memoir; it is hard science beautifully translated; it is funny; it is intersectional; it will crack you open and fill you with awe. Required reading for mothers, and double-required for everyone else."

—Lindy West, author of *New York Times* bestseller *Shrill: Notes from a Loud Woman*

"You don't have to be a mother or even a woman to be fascinated by the science and physiology that Garbes writes about."

—NPR's *Fresh Air*

"*Like a Mother* is the evidence-based, open-minded book that U.S. pregnancy culture needs. . . . A true feminist accomplishment that puts trust and agency back with women and parents."

—Rewire News Group

"An empowering resource. . . . Garbes shares up-to-date, well-substantiated information about women's physical and mental health, aiming to help readers reduce their anxiety and make truly informed choices."

—*Publishers Weekly*

"*Like a Mother* illustrates scientific fact with frankness and intimate detail."

—*New York* magazine

"The science is sublime. I especially appreciated, oddly, learning how much we still don't know about the high-stakes path to parenthood. But what got me was Garbes's regard for mothers as people in their own right, rather than the hosts or self-sacrificing caregivers they're conditioned to be."

—*Seattle Times*

"The pregnancy book that every smart feminist woman has been waiting for has finally arrived! Garbes's natural curiosity and enthusiasm is infectious and never sacrificed as she navigates the culture of pregnancy and once-taboo subjects like miscarriage, placentas, and the pelvic floor with humor and delight. Garbes insists, rightly and beautifully, that women deserve more: more information, more compassion, more autonomy, as well as more support. I read *Like a Mother* in one sitting, and read half of it out loud to my husband. I finished the book filled with hope and gratitude, convinced that this book is both necessary and long overdue."

—Meaghan O'Connell, author of *And Now We Have Everything*

ESSENTIAL
LABOR

ALSO BY ANGELA GARBES

Like a Mother

ESSENTIAL
LABOR

Mothering as
Social Change

ANGELA GARBES

HARPER WAVE

An Imprint of HarperCollins*Publishers*

HarperCollins books may be purchased for educational, business, or sales promotional use. For information, please email the Special Markets Department at SPsales@harpercollins.com.

FIRST EDITION

Designed by Bonni Leon-Berman

Library of Congress Cataloging-in-Publication Data has been applied for.

ISBN 978-0-06-293736-0

22 23 24 25 26   LSC   10 9 8 7 6 5 4 3 2 1

For all my siblings in diasporic feels

I am trying to invent a new way of moving under my
dress: the room squares off against this

—*C. D. Wright*

CONTENTS

INTRODUCTION

WHEN ASKED TO DESCRIBE MY mother I've often said, "She's a natural-born caretaker." It wasn't an answer I thought about deeply; it was simply that every story I heard about her, everything I observed in my childhood, made it clear. As a girl growing up in Mandaluyong, one of sixteen cities that make up the crowded Metro Manila area, she found a frail chick in the courtyard of her family's house. The bird was small and bedraggled, its feathers dirty, and it had trouble walking. She vowed to nurse it back to health—feeding, stroking, and tucking it into her bed at night. Eventually, the bird recovered, and she decided to keep it as her pet. One morning she woke to find it lifeless. She was devastated when she realized that, deep in sleep, she had rolled over and suffocated her beloved bird.

This early tragedy didn't deter my mother from pursuing a career caring for others. Nursing was a relatively new but flourishing career option for Pinay women in the 1960s, and she decided to become a registered nurse, training at Philippine General Hospital before immigrating to the United States. For the majority of her career in America she worked as a hospice nurse, driving to people's homes to care for them during their last stages of life. By the time she met her patients, death was imminent. She administered medications, bathed them, drew blood, communicated with doctors, rotated bodies to provide relief from bedsores, and sat with loved ones. She often worked thirteen-hour days and grew intimately close to these families. To this day, she receives Christmas cards from some of the people she served.

I experienced the power of her caregiving as her child, but also as someone who saw what she did in the world, how much other people appreciated her. At times, she told me recently, she felt more valued by her patients' families than her own. Shame flooded my system as she said it, because I know that in my youth I barely acknowledged the labor she put into our family.

It took being pregnant with my first child to start considering the care I took for granted. How had I felt but never really understood the roughness of my mother's hands, callused and cracked from so much hand and dish washing? How did she raise three children while working full-time? How had I forgotten, until I found myself doing it, the way she slapped her cheeks with one hand, the other on the steering wheel, to stay awake while driving? One of the luxuries of my childhood was to remain oblivious to all the work that went into raising me.

My parents wanted to protect their children from having to think about the complexities of the world, particularly its cruelties. Each fluent in two or more languages, they chose to raise me to speak only English. It wasn't until I was a teenager, pushing the issue, that my father finally admitted their decision wasn't based on my unwillingness to learn Tagalog, as he had once claimed, but instead his refusal to subject his children to the discrimination he endured because of his accent. I sometimes feel they did me a disservice by not passing the language on to me. Whatever anger I feel, though, is abated by my own guilt over never having mastered Tagalog. Of speaking better Spanish, which I learned in high school, than our native tongue.

I heard Tagalog spoken every day; I've never believed English should be the language everyone in America speaks. I've loved Filipino food since I was a child, only ever wanted to eat more, try more, to understand its roots and ingredients—from China, Spain, Mexico. I've been obsessed with being able to identify Filipinx people wherever I go, priding myself on just being able to look at them—a bridgeless nose, a point with the lips, a certain wideness of the cheeks—and intuiting that they are one of my people. I honed these skills during a childhood spent searching faces and names, desperate to find anyone like me.

I was curious about who I was—who I *really* was. I was hungry, desirous of my Filipina identity. More so, it seemed, than my two older brothers. I've been collecting clues and mining information all my life: from recipes, immigration stories, books, figuring out who the men on Philippine pesos—Ninoy Aquino, Emilio Aguinaldo—were, piecing together a trail of crumbs.

At times, my parents were reticent to answer my questions. Now, as we get older, information flows more easily. Now, I ask more questions. I take the time to really listen.

In turn, they begin to be open to what I have to say, the history I've found in books and in conversations with other first-generation Filipinx Americans. We can all see our story as part of a larger one, one that is sometimes painful, one that sometimes threatens to erase their individual triumphs. We're no longer talking at or through each other. Finally, we are in conversation.

MY PARENTS MIGRATED TO THE United States in 1971, just after earning their nursing and medical degrees at the University of the Philippines. Eventually they settled in rural central Pennsylvania, where my brothers and I grew up. Our small town was almost entirely white. Each fall, the first day of deer hunting season meant we got the day off from school.

The first thing I knew about my father's life outside of our home was that "he takes care of dead people"—or at least this is what a slightly dismayed preschool teacher relayed to my parents the day I shared the information at circle time. My father, more accurately, is a pathologist who performed the occasional autopsy, dissecting a body to discern what caused a person's death. In reality he spent most of his days peering through a microscope, searching thin glass slides smeared with tissue samples for cell irregularities, diagnosing disease. I wanted to be able to look at things the way he did, see the hidden things that only he saw. Though they didn't capture my childhood imagination the way cadavers did, I thought the slides were beautiful, stained gradations of pink and purple unfurling like nebulae in space.

My parents worked hard. They were both good at their jobs. They quickly ascended from new immigrants with very little to homeowners with savings. In many ways, we were a typical middle-class American family. My parents could afford to send us to a private Catholic elementary school. They were thrifty; I remember regular trips to a store called the Cannery, where my mom bought dented cans of generic brand soup. But we lacked nothing. We ate dinner together every night, mostly Filipino food like sinigang and adobo, but also stir-fries and Old El Paso hard-shell tacos (my favorite). Despite the outward signs of success, I saw how their adaptability, even their exceptionalism, couldn't protect them from small, lancing indignities such as being condescended to socially and professionally, having their accents mocked, their competency questioned, and their food looked at askance. For as long as I can remember, though we never spoke of it, I was aware that we existed outside of things: respectable but always on the edge of acceptance.

As the poet Cathy Park Hong writes, "one characteristic of racism is that children are treated like adults and adults are treated like children. . . . To grow up Asian in America is to witness the humiliation of authority figures like your parents."[1]

As a child I didn't have the capacity to name what my parents experienced as racism, but I can instantly recall the confusion it caused me. I was embarrassed both by and for them, how they weren't able to hide the alien parts of themselves, how they made me foreign and weird by association. I was angry that they could be degraded so easily, often by people who I understood to be common, basic, uninteresting. I wanted to defend them as much as I wanted to hide and disappear. Mostly, I wanted to translate the world we lived in for them: tell them how to get by unnoticed, explain to white people that they were normal, smart, and funny.

I approached everything slightly sideways, eyes open and observant, head tilted: distrustful, ready to be defensive or feign indifference to those around me. As I grew up, I felt myself to be made of irreconcilable layers and parts. Being the child of immigrants gave me a sort of double consciousness, which, while exhausting, led to a distinct perspective. I can't help but always try to sense things from multiple points of view. I am always trying to protect and safeguard our dignity.

What my mother and father did, day in and day out, illuminated my body's many needs and vulnerabilities. The bodies my parents cared for were the backdrop of our lives. The simple question "How was your day?" was typically answered with stories of ailments, demise, recovery, survival. Their work democratized human bodies, made care part of everyday life and conversation. I consider this my most valuable inheritance, one that I hope to pass down to my own children.

IN MANY WAYS, FILIPINX PEOPLE are the care workers of the world.

Since the mid-1960s, the Philippines has made human labor its greatest export. Each year, more than two million Filipinos leave their homeland. About one in seven Filipinos works abroad, and the $32 billion that these overseas foreign workers (or OFW, as they are commonly called) send back accounts for 10 percent of the country's gross domestic product.[2]

Between 1965 and 1988, more than seventy thousand foreign nurses entered the United States, the majority coming from countries throughout Asia. The Philippines is by far the leading supplier of nurses to America. Paul Ong and Tania Azores estimate that at least twenty-five thousand Filipino nurses migrated to the United States between 1966 and 1985, arguing that a discussion of immigrant Asian nurses, of foreign-trained nurses in general, is "predominantly about Filipino nurses."[3]

Approximately one in four working Filipinx adults are frontline health-care workers.[4] In California, almost 20 percent of RNs are Filipinx.[5] Additionally, because these nurses are more likely to work in ICU nursing and acute care, since March 2020 they are most likely to care for Covid-19 patients.

Thanks to my parents, care work is always at the top of my mind, the underlying force that sustains our lives. It is no longer something I take for granted, certainly not now that I am the mother of two children.

During this long season of pandemic living, I recommitted myself to care work. Because there was so much of it to do, yes, but also because what, each day, could I actually control? I couldn't stop a racist president from telling the country that "Kung Flu" and the "China Virus" would just go away. My daughters and I could send posthumous birthday cards to Breonna Taylor via the Kentucky attorney general's office, but I couldn't make him charge the officers who killed her with murder. I might feel some relief that we were driving less and lowering climate emissions; I could not stop wildfires from consuming the West Coast, choking the air black, and keeping us inside our homes, coughing, for weeks.

But, I could ask: Would you like oatmeal for breakfast? Do you have to go potty? Are you sure? Are you having a big feeling? Do you want to tell me about it? Do you need a snack? Do you need a hug? These questions were the foreground of my mornings, afternoons, and evenings—and they were of vital significance. A good day could grind to a halt if blood sugar crashed or a feeling went unaddressed, only to assert itself later in the form of a tantrum. The smallest details became of the utmost importance.

Early on in quarantine, I found myself thinking, "What is the most valuable thing I could be doing with my time?" The answer clearly wasn't writing an article or making a podcast, but rather keeping my family, and my community, safe and healthy. It is an honor to care for them; they are parts and extensions of myself.

AFTER PUBLISHING MY FIRST BOOK, about the science and culture of pregnancy, I wanted to move away from writing about motherhood. I know it's a subject relevant to everyone, but I bristled at the way "mom books," whether they are fiction, advice books, nonfiction, or memoir, tend to get lumped together and covered generically as a timely trend or topic. I resisted being pigeonholed in a genre that many consider niche. Mother is just one aspect of my identity.

I learned a lot writing my book, but I've learned even more since. The terrain of mothering is not limited to the people who give birth to children; it is not defined by gender. While "mother" is an important identity for many women who still provide the majority of care to children in America, no one cares for children entirely on their own. My perspective has grown to consider the work of raising children as *mothering*, an action that includes people of all genders and nonparents alike. I think of my daughters' bilingual preschool teachers, native Spanish speakers who have instilled values of community responsibility in them, while always encouraging joy and play. There is my mother, who is a regular and beloved presence in their lives. I am grateful for our babysitter Penelope, now twenty years old, who has been caring for our girls since before she could drive. And, over the last two years, I came to rely on my friends Becca and Jondou, our "pod" co-parents, who care for my children as though they are their own, and for whose two children I hold an affection I thought was reserved for my daughters.

I owe this understanding to writers and thinkers including Dani McClain, whose book *We Live for the We: The Political Power of Black Motherhood* inspired me to reread the anthology *Revolutionary Mothering*, edited by Alexis Pauline Gumbs, China Martens, and Mai'a Williams. Rather than viewing care work as characteristic of the noun "motherhood," I now see it as the action of *mothering*, which includes anyone who is engaged in "the practice of creating, nurturing, affirming and supporting life."[6]

What these people cemented in me is the fact that raising

children is not a private hobby, not an individual duty. It is a social responsibility, one that requires robust community support. The pandemic revealed that mothering is some of the only truly essential work humans do. Without people to care for our children, we are lost. Writing about mothering—right now—is more consequential than ever.

Mothering is hard work. It's mentally, physically, and emotionally exhausting. For millions of Americans, the home is where the real work—the work that never changes, never stops, never goes away—gets done. Weekends aren't time off for parents; they are two long days of caregiving.

American society values work in terms of how much we produce, and how efficiently we can do it. It tells us that our output is our worth. Caregiving, conversely, is inefficient. But it pays dividends. If we were to think about work in terms of our humanity—making people feel dignified, valued, and whole—then caregiving is the most important work we can do with our time on earth.

When you become a mother, you engender life, endless possibilities. Mothering is creative in a very literal sense—it is cultivating all that potential, bringing a small person into consciousness. In the pandemic, even as I mourned the loss of the creative outlet of my writing, I discovered that my best moments of mothering happen when I redirect my energy and come to my children with a sense of play and curiosity. It happens in my body—when I get down on all fours and meow with my toddler, as well as my mind, when I think of the truest, most age-appropriate way to answer my seven-year-old, a new reader who recites every condiment label out loud, when she asks, "What's a GMO?"

IN A SOCIETY THAT STILL believes a "normal" person to be a cis, straight white man, so many of us are made to feel that we are, in some way or another, anomalies. But this is simply untrue. As caregivers, we can affirm each child's existence, praise them for their uniqueness, celebrate their idiosyncrasies. When children are greeted with such acceptance, they are likely to be more accepting and tolerant themselves. But they need to be taught, actively. Mothers and caregivers are our first teachers.

"Enormous reversals and revisions of our thinking patterns will have to be achieved somehow, and fast. And to accomplish such lifesaving alterations of society, we will have to deal with power: we will have to make love powerful," the poet June Jordan wrote in 1977.[7]

The urgency Jordan insisted upon still applies. How might our world be different if, from the beginning of life, we were taught that our bodies are nothing less than glorious; that we are enough exactly as we are; that all people, no matter what they look like, are deserving of love, pleasure, and ease?

During the pandemic, I witnessed all my wild, racing thoughts and frustrations about the state of caregiving in America showing up in newspapers, on television, and in Zoom conversations. As I saw how many other people were talking about this issue, I felt a need for us to take advantage of this moment, to blow the conversation open, invite in new perspectives, and imagine new possibilities. Doing this requires knowledge of the history of mothering and care work—how they came to be seen as naturally female, which is to say invisible and undervalued. When we understand the origins of this predicament, we can not only reject it, but offer better, more equitable solutions in its place. We can finally, properly acknowledge the role of care in our society and honor its place in all of our lives. It is time to double down on the radical power of mothering.

In the first part of this book, I explore how we got to where we are today: a wealthy country with an invaluable force of women, most of them brown and Black, performing our most important work for free or at poverty wages. The history is long and complicated, so I am grounding it in what I know best: my own family's story, a story of gendered and racialized care beginning in the Philippines and set in motion by American imperial force. I place mothering in a global and national context of care—the invisible economic engine that has been historically demanded of women of color. I highlight commonalities with other laborers, and opportunities for solidarity among mothers, caregivers, and domestic workers.

In the second part of the book, I dwell in the details of caregiving; the small decisions that make up each day, reminding us of the weight they carry, how their importance accumulates to become a major force in our children's lives. Mothering means tending to children's physical needs, which is where we can begin teaching them progressive, inclusive,

freedom- and pleasure-centered ways of understanding human bodies and their places in the world.

To be clear, I don't know what I'm doing. I'm making up
my parenting as I go along, unlearning so much of what I've
been taught or assumed for much of my life, and trying to figure out what and how, exactly, to teach my children. Drawing
from my own questions, mistakes, experiences, and research,
I offer space to reimagine the chores that often seem overwhelming and laborious as opportunities to craft meaning
and—this is the dream—contribute to positive social change.

"Everyday life is the primary terrain of social change,"
writes Silvia Federici, one of the founders of Wages for
Housework, an international grassroots campaign formed in
1972 to demand payment for care work. The repetitive tasks
of mothering—wiping butts, cleaning food off the floor, reading books over and over, keeping track of clothes that are on
the verge of being outgrown—constitute everyday life. This is
essential work that makes all other work possible. It is vital to
the economy, yet it is underpaid, if compensated at all.

What I have found working in the home is a profoundly satisfying way to be of use. In these strange and difficult years of
instability, loss, and grief—both general and intimate—I've
learned that showing up every day and doing something real,
however small, is the best thing you can do. Each day spent
with children offers so many opportunities to shape a more
caring and equitable world.

For years, I've been asking myself the same question over
and over: How, under our current circumstances that leave
mothers and caregivers so depleted, might we demand more

from American family life? Raising children should not be as lonely, bankrupting, and exhausting as it is. While we must demand recognition and remuneration for care work, we can't afford to wait around for governmental support. Our needs are urgent.

Reimagining our approach to mothering can birth its transformative potential. Day in and day out, this work can be our most consistent, embodied resistance to patriarchy, white supremacy, ableism, and the exploitation that underlies American capitalism. I think of the bodies that my parents cared for—bodies that provided for us, gave me a safe and comfortable upbringing. I want to give all bodies—brown, Black, disabled, queer—the attention and tenderness we deserve but that this country has never granted us.

"The aim of each thing we do is to make our lives and the lives of our children richer and more possible," writes Audre Lorde.[8] I love her directive for both its vagueness and expansiveness. It calls on each of us to take stock of our priorities, to get creative with what we know we can do, with the belief that our actions take root in our children and we can grow the world we want starting right now.

Love and care, like social change, are slow and follow circuitous paths—they take days not hours, years not months. The work may seem inefficient, but love doesn't play by the same rules as the economy. The economy could stand to bend to the will of decency and care. What if we built a system that lets us actually care for the people who care for us? When we are parenting from within, feeling confident and secure in our bodies, rooted in pleasure and love, we are better able to meet the goals Lorde set forth. Embodied mothering, which leads to embodied children who become the next generation of adults, can be our best offense and defense against the inhumane, distinctly American lifestyle.

Raising a child requires profound strength and hope. You must believe in your ability to forge a future that is better than the present we currently inhabit, even if you never live to see it. We should think of ourselves as actively raising people who will never think less of someone based on the shape of their body or the color of their skin; who will feel as welcome in the forest as they do at the head of a table; who understand that their lives are intimately tied to the lives of others; who have full body autonomy. We are raising future community members and leaders—adults who will never put children in cages, never ask someone to choose between their health and a paycheck.

Nearly every adult—let alone parent—I know has talked about having to reckon with, and unlearn, values and rules that they were taught as children. For many women, the importance of taking up as little space as possible and putting other people's needs before your own. For men, the idea that showing emotion is a sign of weakness. For both, that vulnerability and interdependence are bad. We see now that this way of living does not lead to our health and well-being, as individuals and a society.

I reject silver-lining approaches to the pandemic because there is just too much loss and grief to ignore. But I am interested in what can be taken from it, what it has revealed, how these truths might change us and our perspective. When I

We restructure and rearrange the way we live, how we define our lives, and what we value.

The Filipinx culture writer Ligaya Mishan observes that, "When you are raised in two cultures at once—when people see in you two heritages at odds, unresolved, in abeyance—you learn to shift at will between them. You may never feel like you quite belong in either, but neither are you fully constrained."[9]

Mishan is writing about first-generation kids like myself, kids of immigrants, but I think many of us now—particularly white people finally awake to their privilege but unsure what, exactly, to do with that—can relate. We are caught between how we were raised and how we really want to live. We should feel free rather than limited. Free to try new ways of supporting families, free to possibly fail. Free to, as the kids say, "fuck around and find out." We need everyone, and there's no better time to start than right now.

There is a tension to parenting, between the vast possibilities you work toward and the limits of what we caregivers can do. Children grow up, and a necessary part of maturation is moving away from family, developing independent thinking. There are no guarantees.

I am nothing like my parents and yet I am everything like them. I absorbed what they taught me, but the American and global cultural landscape that I was raised in has formed me too. My life and identity have grown far beyond what my parents pictured for me—into a distinct sense of self that I have forged from my own will and ambition. As a Filipinx American, I am acutely aware of how my life differs from that of my parents. But as a first-generation Fil Am, I also identify strongly with my mother and father, the first of their families to step into uncertainty and make their own path. We are all trailblazers in our own ways. Now I look to the leadership of younger people. I see how my daughters, mixed-race Filipina American white Czech Germans, will be the first of their kind too—growing up in a digital, burning world that is constantly being made and remade and pushed forward. Now my vision stretches beyond me and into the future, into what sort of world our children will exist and, hopefully, be free and thrive in.

My daughters are young, and I know that my influence over them is still the dominant force in their lives. It hurts to admit that I find myself thinking of the outside world, American culture, with fear—as dogs coming to nip at their heels, snatch their confidence with bared incisors, the full force of institutions behind those sharp teeth. I want to believe that what I teach them will stick, what I model for them will last. The truth is, I don't know. But I am certain that if I don't at least try, they will never know the full potential of their lives.

Let's let it rip, go hard in the paint, let it all hang out. Let's raise our children as well as we can, together. Let's instill in them deeply rooted, undeniable, impenetrable, unshakeable beliefs in their own worth, their right to liberation and to feel pleasure in their bodies, to see themselves as inextricably linked to other humans, all other life on earth.

Let's raise our children to know these things in their bones and cells, their meat and marrow, have it be part of them. For that understanding to be so strong that it cannot be undone by the colonial and capitalist systems that will insist their worth is how much they can produce, how thin their bodies are, how dedicated to work they are. So strong that instead these systems will crumble in the face of young people who—simply by existing, joyfully and fully—insist on a better world.

PART I

A PERSONAL HISTORY OF MOTHERING IN AMERICA

The only way to survive is by taking care of one another.

—GRACE LEE BOGGS

1

MOTHERING
AS SURVIVAL

In March 2020, my daughters, five and two at the time, went to preschool every day. Our days began at 6:30 a.m. in a noisy, chaotic swirl of coffee grinding, diaper changing, egg frying, oatmeal simmering, dressing, undressing, crying, and re-dressing, shoelace tying, and coat zipping-up. In the wake, toys were left scattered across the living room and maple syrup stuck to the dining room table. My spouse dropped our kids off on his way to the office, though, so having doled out kisses and hugs by the front door, I was typically alone by 8:15. I enjoyed the silence, wondered how it was that I could feel so tired so early in the day. Then I'd head upstairs to our guest room, aka "my office," where I worked on a book that I had been (mostly unsuccessfully) trying to write for two years.

Then the Covid-19 pandemic began. Lockdown changed the world and daily life as we knew it. Childcare centers, schools, offices, libraries, coffee shops, and friends' homes closed to all of us overnight and indefinitely.

For the next four months, our family of four was together 24/7, mostly within the walls of our home. We knew little about the virus and how it was contracted, so we followed the advice we were given: we disinfected our groceries, washed and sanitized our hands until they were red and peeling. We went on daily walks and scooter rides during which the children instinctively led us to neighborhood parks where the swing sets and play structures stood ghostly empty, wrapped in yellow Caution tape. There were so many hours to fill each day, so much need, so much *us*.

During those early months, my daughters' requirements were seemingly constant: three meals a day (plus snacks, always snacks), hours for physical play, piles of books to read aloud, at least four diaper changes. We did so much vulva and butt wiping those months that we vowed to turn quarantine summer into the season of potty training. During those months I was overwhelmed and clinically depressed, but things needed to get done. The kitchen sink was perpetually full of dishes; the laundry mountain grew every day.

My spouse and I know our professional work to be equally important. We spend an annoying amount of our time in logistical negotiations, discussing how to split domestic work equitably. Yet our new reality made clear the fact that my work, with its deadlines on the distant horizon, doesn't provide us with a regular paycheck or health insurance. If I didn't show up to my desk to write, no one would know—there were no consequences outside of my own psyche. But if my spouse failed to show up to the makeshift office he set up in our garage, the Uber, Lyft, and taxi drivers he was working with—mostly East African immigrants, nearly all of whom were suddenly out of work because no one was going anywhere—might not be able to access unemployment benefits. The results would be dire.

I am a woman of color, a writer, a mother. I don't like the very gendered fact that I am dependent on my white husband's salary, and I worry that it may take me a lifetime to undo the false notion that my work is somehow less valuable than his. Added to this long-standing issue was now the unfortunate fact that I could not seem to write anything during quarantine. It was impossible, without time and space and solitude, to get into the already elusive headspace I need to do deep, creative work.

In the fall of 2020, a *New York Times* survey found that among heterosexual couples working from home during the pandemic, men were more likely than women to work in a separate room or home office. "Women," wrote Claire Cain Miller, "were more likely to work at the kitchen table, where they could be interrupted at any moment by children or household needs."[1]

My husband and I tag-team parented, a few hours on, a few hours off, a few hours together. When it was my turn to work, I closed the door to our guest bedroom and stared blankly at my computer screen, trying not to check daily infection rates. Inevitably, a child would breach the only two things protecting my solitude: the guest room door and a pair of noise-canceling headphones. It was inconceivable that I could write for one hour without disruption.

"More than in any other human relationship, overwhelmingly more, motherhood means being instantly interruptible," wrote Tillie Olsen in 1968. "It is distraction, not meditation, that becomes habitual; interruption, not continuity."[2]

Women are not innately better at caregiving than men. I am not more inclined or effective at it than my husband. What I found most troubling was realizing that I was the one allowing interruption to be habitual. That, it turns out, I had a hard time insisting upon my own time and space.

I took care of my daughters, shouldered a heavier load of domestic work, and tried to continue my writing—all while feeling that doing any of it well was impossible. Daily anxieties played out against the backdrop of America's rising death toll, skyrocketing unemployment numbers, continued broadcast of murders of Black men and women and children, and climate crises that turned once sweltering states into surreal sheets of ice. As spring gave way to summer, we came back outside to meet our neighbors in the streets and protest. Walking in the sticky heat of the sun, among the bodies we'd been away from for so long, my emotions swelled with grief and fear that our country's habits would never change.

I HAVE A NICE LIFE, one my parents say was made possible by the American Dream. But I am an American because of American imperialism.

My introduction to empire came in childhood, helping my mother pack and label balikbayan boxes for a trip back to the Philippines. Each member of our family was allotted two pieces of checked baggage; all children were expected to surrender at least one to a balikbayan box the size of the maximum space allowed by the airline. The balikbayan operation, which took over our living room for weeks, was one I had observed for years. I was thrilled to finally join the ritual, Tetris-like packing of enormous cardboard cubes filled with Reese's Pieces, Nike sneakers, three-packs of Hane's men's briefs, boxes of Ziploc bags, Ferrero Rocher chocolates, and other items. All the gifts were crammed in amid hundreds of face towels and washcloths, bought in bulk at whatever department store had recently had a linen sale and exclusively for my paternal grandmother Ima, who sold them for profit at the supermarket she owned. The pasalubong was expected, my mom explained, given out of love and the financial success my parents had achieved abroad. At the time, I took it to mean we were giving our less fortunate Filipino relatives the American goods they could not afford otherwise.

After being filled and weighed, each balikbayan box was sealed and wrapped in packing tape, the screeching sound and chemical plastic smell of which filled the house. Cages of bright yellow or pink twine—for easy identification amid the sea of other boxes at baggage claim as well as easy lifting from the carousel—were knotted around them. Then our family name and address were written in foul-smelling black Sharpie on four sides of each box: Garbes Dizon Supermarket, MacArthur Highway, San Fernando, Pampanga. The road my grandparents lived and worked on is named after the American general whose decisions led to so much Philippine death and heartache during World War II.

I learned and memorized the proper spelling of the Philippines through labeling balikbayan boxes until my hand ached. It was an object lesson in the lasting effects of colonialism.

"Write PHILIP for the King of Spain," my mom instructed me. "Then PINES, like the trees outside." I found Spain on our globe afterward, unsure why our country on the other side of the world would be named for its king. Later I learned that in 1544, Spanish explorer Ruy López de Villalobos, having sailed across the Pacific from Mexico, claimed and named a few islands for his king. Eventually, this archipelago—comprised of more than seven thousand islands and over one hundred Indigenous ethnic groups with their own customs and languages—would be condensed into one country, now known as the Philippines.

YOU CAN SAY THAT MY parents came to America for a better life, and that they got one. In fact, they would be the first ones to say so. But that tidy narrative oversimplifies the story and fails to capture the geopolitical manipulations that shaped their paths.

My parents met in 1969 at Manila's Philippine General Hospital. My mom was a quiet twenty-two-year-old nurse who kept her hair slicked neatly back in a ponytail at the nape of her neck; my dad was a medical student with a perpetually wrinkled lab coat, big lips, and a head of wild curls. My mom says her first impression of him was that he was a "slob." Six months later they were married.

As the seventh of nine children, my mom was told that upon graduation she would work as a nurse in the United States and send money home to help her two younger sisters go to college. My father, the eldest of seven and the first person in his family to attend college, was instructed to study a profession he was expected to pursue for the rest of his life. Though my parents were not aware of it at the time, their decisions to work in health care and move to the United States were shaped and constrained by centuries of conquest, bloodshed, and American policy.

Prior to the passing of the US Immigration Act of 1965, also known as the Hart-Celler Act, which lifted quotas on visas for skilled workers from other countries, Filipino migration had been limited to just fifty visas a year. This was the lowest number allotted to any country in the world, a harsh reversal from the previous decades when Filipinos, called "U.S. Nationals" under American colonial rule, were able to travel freely throughout the United States and its territories. Filipino bodies—hands, backs, knees, minds, voices—have always been viewed as economic leverage for the United States.

The US government's decision to allow an influx of Filipino workers such as my mother conveniently coincided with a nursing shortage in the United States. In the two decades following World War II, the rapid growth of hospitals, higher demand for health-care services, and creation of medical insurance made filling nursing positions across the country difficult. While hospital managers believed the shortage was caused by women leaving the workforce to care for their families, nurses stated that low wages and poor working conditions were to blame. They organized and advocated for better pay, but efforts stalled as nurses held little status within hospitals, and administrators opted to hire supporting workers—nurse aides and practical nurses, rather than registered nurses.[3] Recruiting and bringing in a skilled foreign labor force, aided by the Hart-Celler Act, allowed hospital administrators to keep costs low.

My mother, a graduate of the colonial education system who spoke fluent English and held a brand-new nursing degree, qualified for immigration in 1970. My father, who never intended to leave the Philippines, reluctantly agreed to move to America for love. His medical degree made obtaining a visa relatively easy. My mother followed the path of many Filipina nurses before her—and tens of thousands after.

"Her story is a part of something larger, it is a part / of history," poet Rick Barot writes of his grandmother's journey from the Philippines to the United States many years before. With these words, I can grasp the magnitude of forces that sent my mother across the Pacific.

"Or, no, her story is separate / from the whole, as distinct as each person is distinct," Barot goes on, and I see my mother—a brave individual in a foreign country, with a new husband, and a burgeoning sense of self—forging her way forward.

"Or, her story / is surrounded by history, the ambient spaciousness / of which she is the momentary foreground," continues Barot.[4] I now see my mother's story as her own, important and distinct, but always part of a larger diasporic whole that I will spend my life trying to wrap my mind and heart around.

IN THE PHILIPPINES, THE UNITED STATES essentially created a farming ground, a steady and growing supply of health-care workers. The workforce, primarily Filipino nurses, was also decidedly gendered and racialized—female and brown.

The understanding of the wave of Filipina nurses who immigrated to America after 1965 is often framed solely in terms of the quotas lifted by Hart-Celler. But in this simplified version, historian Catherine Ceniza Choy notes, "rendered invisible are the ways U.S. hospital recruiters have collaborated across national boundaries with Philippine travel and recruitment agencies in their aggressive recruitment of Filipino nurses." Ceniza Choy cites the work of Jon Goss and Bruce Lindquist, who call this practice the *institutionalization of migration*.[5]

Within this institutional framework, problems such as the exploitation of Filipina nurses by Philippine and American recruiters, as well as American hospitals, are erased from the story. So, too, are accounts of white women's animosity toward Filipinx nurses. History purposely obscures ugly realities that, for different reasons, both Americans and Filipinos would prefer to forget. The truth, ever more complicated, is that these stories are painful for people to recount, especially those raised to worship the country they migrate to and be thankful for any opportunities given to them. And so, for the

sake of not making a fuss, many immigrants willingly pro-
mote the narrative of coming to America simply for financial
promise.

While my parents earned more money in the United States
than they would have back home, they were on their own
without any support, overwhelmed, and made to feel out of
place. My mom often took double shifts when my father was
working because she couldn't bear to be home alone.

There wasn't room in the house I grew up in for existential
worry. Life's difficulties were spoken about matter-of-factly,
items to cross off a to-do list. I remember being a teenager
at the dining room table when Dr. Jack Kevorkian dominated
the news. My mother, a devout pro-life Catholic, looked at
me and said, "When it's my time, no heroics, *you let me die.*"
For all their frank talk about disease and death, though, my
parents never talked to me about the obvious realities of our
bodies—how we were different from others in our community, how that might affect our emotions, our sense of selves.
These are precisely the conversations I craved and the conversations I pursue now.

My parents never spoke openly about our bodies because
of their cultural inheritance. They came from a country colonized first by Spain and the Catholic Church, and then by
the United States. Subservience, an idea of being less than, of
equating being good and acceptable with being indistinguish-
able and assimilated, smooth rather than resistant, were
what they were taught. But probing my parents, pushing my
mother past the easy answer of "a better life," reveals more

ambivalence and complication. Both she and my father were actively recruited to emigrate. They were fronted money by agencies and hospitals for their airfare, which was later deducted from their early paychecks.

When I ask about this, my dad initially insists that their situation was really no different from other American nurses and medical students who might have had to pay back student loans. But when I point out that the high cost of medical school in the States makes it so that most people who pursue it are white and come from economic privilege, he agrees. As we talk further, he concedes that it is easier to be taken advantage of or exploited by people who claim to be helping you.

My father takes pride in having come here with nothing and having worked his way into the middle class against the expectations of many people he encountered. Eventually he secured a place in the upper middle class, where he can now buy substantial things, say a car or a trip for our whole family, whenever he wants. It's important to him that he has earned this position—and he doesn't think he should have to tamp down his whims for anything.

My husband grew up in a much harder economic situation; these spending habits were completely out of the realm of consideration for his family After the birth of our first child, each time my parents visited—on a random Monday or weekend—they brought a gift. They like to make every day feel like a special occasion. It made us uncomfortable; we didn't need more stuff. Will and I decided to talk to them—

and thought it would be better if he led the conversation. So, one day, they sat down, and he explained that he grew up with very little, that getting a gift was a big deal, a truly memorable event, and that we'd prefer it if they would consult with us in advance and save their generosity for holidays and birthdays. My mother started crying and said, "If you think there is someone else who is better suited for caring for your daughter than me, then maybe you should go ahead and hire them." My father stood up from the couch and looked Will square in the eye: "I hear what you are saying. And I totally disagree. I came to this country with nothing and now I can buy whatever I want. Nothing and no one will stop me from buying any gift for my granddaughter that I want to, whenever I feel like it."

My father knows that the relationship between the United States and the Philippines—the relationship that made his comfortable life possible—is inherently an exploitative one. After a few moments of silence in our conversation he said, "Sometimes I think that the best thing that ever could have happened to the Philippines is that they made it a state, like Hawaii. Then life there would be better than it is now."

It occurs to me he might be articulating something that he has felt for years, decades even, but never said out loud. I think of a line from Elaine Castillo's novel *America Is Not the Heart*: "Baggage means no matter how far you go, no matter how many times you immigrate, there are countries in you you'll never leave."[6]

In this moment I see how deep colonialism runs, how fully it penetrates the psyche. For years my father has thought the solution to being colonized would be to be "saved" by the colonizers. It's a cruel trick, its long-lasting effect devastating to me.

But who am I to judge? I worry I am condescending to him. I get to critique colonization and argue from a position of privilege, having grown up in America, having graduated from college debt-free, the beneficiary of my parents' hard work. I have no idea what it's like to be him, to have lived his life. It's easy to analyze from where I am sitting, to get on a high horse and talk about the colonial mentality, the importance of "decolonizing our minds."

DURING THE EARLY YEARS OF my parents' lives, the Philippines was recovering from the devastation of World War II. The capital city was decimated in the 1945 Battle of Manila, a brutal, month-long Japanese occupation during which soldiers committed mass rape and murder of Filipino civilians, resulting in over one hundred thousand deaths. The US military relentlessly bombed the city, once called the "Pearl of the Orient," as well as its residents, content to regard the destruction of the city and lives as collateral damage. Manila was the second most devastated Allied capital of the war, behind Warsaw.[7] Long after the battle, people remembered the smell of human bodies rotting in the streets.

The United States "acquired" the Philippines, along with Puerto Rico and Guam, from Spain—which had ruled the islands for the previous four hundred years—as a result of its victory in the Spanish-American War in 1898. The Philippines and its people were prizes of conquest from the beginning, though officials recognized that possessing territories went against the American ideals of self-governance and democracy. The United States recast its control of the Philippines as a duty to protect and civilize Filipinos.

"We come not as invokers or conquerors, but as friends, to protect the natives in their homes, in their employments, and in their personal and religious right," President William McKinley told Filipinos in 1898. The mission of the United States was not colonization, he said, but "benevolent assimilation." Those who cooperated with American rule would receive support and protection, but those who preferred not to be assimilated would "be brought within the lawful rule we have assumed, with firmness if need be."[8]

Americans took up "the white man's burden"[9] of civilizing their "little brown brothers" through education and steeping the Filipino people in their cultural ways. They set up English-language public schools modeled after the American system. Because of this, my parents speak English in addition to Tagalog, and my father speaks a third language, his provincial dialect of Kapampangan. The United States also established nursing and medical schools, which they presented as a pathway to economic empowerment for people in a poor country. Among themselves, Americans discussed establishing a medical industry as a way of sanitizing people they saw as inherently backward, dirty, and diseased.[10]

Benevolent assimilation was an effective strategy. Despite the destruction and death caused by both the Japanese and the US military, as a child my father was taught contempt for Japan and reverence for America. Of course he chose to become a doctor.

IN THE HALLWAYS OF HOSPITALS and universities, it was white women who perpetuated the idea that Filipino people needed Americans to become enlightened and proper. Nursing has always been a predominately female field, nurses regarded as assistants to male physicians, and it was white American women who trained Filipinas. While theoretically they were training these women to become their professional equals, American women were repulsed by the thought of having to share dormitory space with Filipinas and to work under their supervision. For white women, the relationship had to be one of dominance.[11]

Since the 1960s, mainstream white American feminism has preached dignity and self-expression through career and work outside the home, a "lean in" approach that values personal growth and gain. These women have had little interest in an inclusive feminism rooted in creating a better society for everyone. While Betty Friedan was publishing *The Feminine Mystique* and advocating for women to find fulfillment through work, the Black, Indigenous, and other leaders of the National Welfare Rights Organization were developing a platform for a universal basic income that improved the lives of all Americans.

White women and men stretched the tentacles of American capitalism and colonialism across the Pacific to the Philippines. They perpetuated a system that allowed the United

States to take what it needed from people when it wanted and shut them out when they preferred not to have them around. These are the same forces that have confined so many Black, Latina, and other Asian women in America to invisible care-taking roles. These women's stories are different, but the reasons behind the power dynamic are the same. Capitalism, patriarchy, and white supremacy have always been at work.

Black and brown women are especially devalued. They are paid less than white women; they are far less represented in positions of power; they are overrepresented in service and care work. Women of color make up 20 percent of the US population, yet they represent 40 percent of all childcare workers. Childcare professionals, many of them mothers, are three times as likely to live in poverty as workers in other professions.[12]

These are the same social, cultural, and colonial forces that set up my mother—a petite, agreeable Filipina woman—to become a professional caregiver, and that would have made it difficult for her to be anything else.

In America, my mother—and tens of thousands of her Filipina peers—found they wanted more than the money they earned. They wanted freedom from the watchful eyes of extended family; they wanted travel and Broadway musicals, grocery stores with frozen and boxed dinners, dishwashers and microwaves, the ability to send boxes of pasalubong back home. In exchange, they were willing to work long hours and unpredictable shifts, and take critical care positions that were more physically demanding and intimate with patients than their white counterparts would accept.[13]

While nursing is a trained and generally respected profession, in the health-care industry nurses are down-and-dirty laborers. They change your bandages, clean your wounds, start IV lines, and bathe you; they tend to your body in ways a physician does not. Nurses are the ones touching you, taking the brunt of your frustration and bad moods, toweling up your fluids, carrying away your body's waste. During the Covid-19 pandemic, the risk of the frontline jobs Filipinx nurses disproportionately occupied—evidence that their lives are considered less valuable than those of white nurses—became devastatingly clear. While Filipina nurses comprise just 4 percent of all the nurses in the United States, they account for 34 percent of nursing deaths from Covid-19.[14]

Look around: loss—personal, public, private, medical, familial, professional—and death is undeniably a part of American daily life right now. It is a crisis that calls for solidarity, especially among women.

Nearly five million jobs have been lost by women during Covid; a significant percentage of women cite childcare as the reason for their unemployment. There are currently two million fewer women in the workforce than there were at the start of 2020. Unemployment hit Black and brown women the hardest, as restaurants, salons, and childcare centers shut down early, some never to reopen. A second wave of labor troubles hit in September 2020, when schools remained closed and 865,000 women left the workforce in a single month because they simply could not perform the roles of teacher, caregiver, and professional worker at the same time.

According to a *New York Times* survey, eight out of ten

mothers managed their children's remote schooling, while seven out of ten are doing the majority of childcare.[15] The pandemic revealed that this can happen to anyone, that work won't save affluent white women, despite Friedan's theorizing. Ultimately, they cannot ever fully outsource domestic labor. It still comes down to them.

As long as the pandemic continues, women will be disproportionately affected by it. What do we lose, exactly, when mothers disappear from the world for a year, or more?

Mothers' work outside the home, whatever form that takes, is directly tied to their participation in public life. American culture has lost so much of our research contributions; writing, music, and creative work; our insights into topics beyond routines and child rearing; our policy ideas. Many mothers, stepmothers, foster mothers, and caregivers do all this work with empathy, with a real understanding of the needs of modern American families: affordable childcare, family leave for all workers, quality health care.

Women out of the workforce, enduring the brunt of economic hardship, is not a short-term problem. Nor is it a recent one. A factor in the gender pay gap is that women, over the course of their careers—mothers or not—will step away from paid work in order to care for family members. They lose money not only in the form of salaries, but also retirement funds and health-care benefits. It takes years to come back fully, often to lower wages. It is destabilizing and demoralizing. At a pandemic scale, it threatens to erase and vanish American women for years, likely decades.

Pandemic living flattened my life and my identity. I could

no longer be the same person out in the world. I began to doubt my own sense of self. For months I secretly wished that my creative impulse, the urge to write, would just die. Then, I thought, I could at least be free of the guilt and shame of wanting more, of being unable to find fulfillment in caring for my family. Then, I reasoned, I could just start over, do any job I wanted—and, preferably, a job that didn't feel so tied to my identity. The white-hot frustration—over dependency on my spouse, the thought that maybe my work really isn't as valuable as his—felt so personal. It was not hard to think there was a flaw in me, that I had made nothing but wrong choices. Each day I fight to remind myself that these are not personal or lifestyle problems, and they are not even pandemic-specific: these are systemic issues that have been built into labor and financial institutions; they are, by design, foundational to American life.

We don't have to choose between a domestic life and a professional one outside the home, nor does fulfillment have to be either/or. It's messy to untangle identity and worth, home and public life, but maybe we can try to allow them to coexist, to find meaning in each of them.

"I appear to need to be alone in order to make things; it appears to be necessary to my survival. And yet my children appear to need me, always; it appears to be necessary for their survival," writes playwright Sarah Ruhl. "And yet for me to feel my sanity, these two practices, of motherhood and making things, so primary, need to feel as though they are compatriots."[16]

Over the last two years, as I've done an unprecedented

amount of caregiving, I've spent an equal amount of time considering care work: how it is seen as low-wage labor, rather than highly skilled work that is essential, creative, and influential. Caregivers know when a child needs a nap, which song sung out loud might calm them. While parents provide these comforts, they also rely on family, friends, childcare workers, babysitters, and nannies. Mothering is the purview of many domestic workers for whom providing quality care means forging familial relationships and acquiring professional knowledge that is sensual and personal.

This expertise lives in the bodies of women of color throughout America. Ninety-two percent of domestic workers are women, and fifty-seven percent of them are Black, Latina, or Asian American/Pacific Islander. We entrust the safety and cleanliness of our homes to Latinx workers, who comprise 62 percent of house cleaners. Whether they mop our floors, care for our elders, or watch our children, there is a wide and long-standing gap between the wages of domestic workers and all other workers in America. While the median wage for workers in this country is nearly twenty dollars an hour, it is barely twelve for domestic workers. The gap is widest for nannies—97 percent of whom are women—who earn a median of just $11.60 an hour. And while the cost of living has steadily risen, the wages of domestic workers have remained mostly stagnant for decades.[17]

We are entrusting that which we say is most precious— our children, our future—to other people, yet we are not willing to pay them a living wage? What does that say about our priorities as a society? About our priorities as individuals? As more people realize how vital this work is, we need to challenge ourselves to properly value and compensate caregivers.

In her 2018 TED talk, Ai-jen Poo, founder and executive director of the National Domestic Workers Alliance (NDWA), encourages us to emulate the many domestic workers who "cross cultures and generations and borders and boundaries" and whose jobs are "to show up and care—to nurture, to feed, to clothe, to bathe, to listen, to encourage, to ensure safety, to support dignity." Whatever hardships they may be facing in their own lives and families, Poo reminds us that every day domestic workers "love and they care, and they show compassion no matter what."[18]

IN THE EARLY, PRE-COVID DAYS of the 2020 presidential election, Elizabeth Warren was seemingly everywhere talking about the challenges of being a working mother, how she couldn't have done it without her Aunt Bea. I remind myself that it was just that summer, during the 2020 Democratic National Convention, that Warren said on national television that childcare is infrastructure—just like roads, bridges, public utilities—for American families.

While working at a law firm, Hillary Clinton crafted her own maternity leave policy because no woman there had ever returned to full-time work after having a child. In 2018, Tammy Duckworth became the first sitting US senator to have a baby while working full-time. I was moved seeing her vote with her newborn in her arms on the Senate floor but also remember thinking: Damn, she deserves more than ten days of leave. We now have a female vice president and the highest ever number of women serving in the House of Representatives and Senate. That record high? Just 27 percent of Congress. The perspective mothers can bring to their jobs—whether it's law making, coalition building, project management—is that family and care work are essential to life, not an inconvenience. Women's labor force participation is currently as low as it was in 1988.[19] What we are losing right now is everything American society has always desperately needed.

Those who truly cannot afford to sit back and wait have continued advocating, organizing, and fighting, even through our darkest recent days. We are seeing shifts in policy and cultural thinking because of them, because they have been working on this issue for decades. Because they have always recognized the value of mothering and the moral obligation of supporting caretakers, we are moving in a positive direction.

Groups such as NDWA have long been organizing domestic workers to campaign for basic labor protections. Since 2010 ten states, including New York, Hawaii, California, Nevada, and Virginia, and two cities, Philadelphia and Seattle, have passed their own domestic workers Bill of Rights to guarantee overtime pay, paid time off, and protections for people subjected to racial or sexual harassment. In July 2021, the New York City Council voted to include domestic workers in the city's Human Rights Law, giving two hundred thousand workers—the majority of whom are women of color—protection from workplace abuse and discrimination.

Before the pandemic, many of us were already navigating

complex choices between our careers and domestic work because the gender pay gap left us with incomes lower than the
cost of childcare. Because the pandemic made outsourcing
care work nearly impossible for everyone, we are now seeing
policy proposals that offer financial support for mothering.

In July 2021, under the Child Tax Credit provision that
is part of the American Rescue Plan, families with children
began receiving monthly direct cash payments. The payments
were slated to amount to $3,000 annually per child up to age
seventeen and $3,600 annually per child under age six. It was
paid to all families, with slightly lower amounts going to people with higher incomes. It was not a perfect plan: it gave less
money to single or unpartnered parents, wrongly assuming
that they have a lower level of expenses and reinforcing the
idea that the nuclear family is the best structure for children.
At the end of 2021, the funding, which was allocated until
July 2022, expired early when Congress failed to renew it.

What if we could make these payments permanent? Putting money directly into the hands of people caring for children is a strong start toward showing parents and caregivers
that we, as a society, value their work. It's hard to imagine
this country committing to funding care. After all, to quote
economists Raj Patel and Jason W. Moore, "to ask for capitalism to pay for care is to call for an end to capitalism."[20] But
isn't now the perfect time to think radically? To get back in
touch with the creativity we've felt so distanced from? Do we
value ourselves enough to try?

Nearly a year after Senator Warren appeared on stage, on
Mother's Day 2021, the headline story of the Business section

of the Sunday *New York Times* read, "How Child Care Became As Essential As Bridges."[21] This signals a massive shift in thinking. Change is happening. How much further we go is up to us. This is an inflection point: a once-in-a-generation moment to invest in the people who mother children, whether bound by blood or affection.

Our stories are our legacy, touched by history and possibility. I inherited my family's story—the limits of their choices, shape of their journey, weight of their baggage, and the generosity of their care. I will pass this down to my daughters. At the height of the pandemic, this country's mothers and essential care workers were in the momentary foreground, but that attention is slipping away. Whether conditions for those who mother improve or stall or regress, we must never stop talking about how we cared—how we continue to care— for one another. Our stories matter; they are how our children will know we survived.

2

MOTHERING AS
VALUABLE LABOR

When my parents immigrated to the United States in 1970, they came alone, with very few belongings. I try to imagine them, just twenty-three and twenty-seven years old, each pursuing someone else's plan for their lives. They had known each other less than a year, and their first home together was a cramped apartment in West Philadelphia, a city whose cold winters were a shock to their sun-warmed systems. My grandmother, Ima, had offered to "send someone" with them: a domestic worker to help with cooking, cleaning, and, eventually, childcare. My dad's family didn't have a lot of money, but in the Philippines having domestic help isn't uncommon, whether or not you are wealthy. My mom declined the offer, which I imagine could not have been easy. Ima, along with my grandfather Tatang, had grown a palengke stand where they bartered imported American goods such as

Marlboros for produce into a corner market, then into a supermarket, and finally a local wholesale market, à la Costco.
Ima birthed seven children and worked at the store seven
days a week until she was one hundred years old. She is a
formidable woman.

"I grew up with maids, Angela," my mother says, dismiss-
ing the idea that it was a difficult decision. "They hear everything you say." She wanted privacy, she says, and she wanted
to be accountable to the family she was building with my father: "Whatever mistakes I made, whatever happens to my
kids, it's my responsibility." She adds that she "didn't want to
be responsible for another person."

My maternal grandfather was a doctor, but, my mom says,
"he wasn't particularly ambitious." Their family of eleven
needed more than just his salary to survive. My maternal
grandmother, Lola Lily, was, in my mom's words, "a hustler
and an entrepreneur." When she fell in love with and married
my grandfather, Lola Lily put her plans to become a doctor
on hold. She channeled that drive into making ends meet—
picking up work as a seamstress, operating a small salon in
her home, crocheting and selling her creations. Eventually,
she opened a pharmacy, taught chemistry on the faculty of
Philippine Women's University, and became the first trea-
surer of the university's credit union.

I remember my Lola as the person who came to our house
every year to hand-sew our Halloween costumes. She had a
lilting voice, played the piano, and loved ballroom dancing.
She also had the softest skin and a hairy blue mole on her

arm, both of which I loved to stroke. She was full of life, vi-
brancy, and warmth. But I didn't know her full story.

"My mother was amazing," my mom says. "But she wasn't
a hands-on, touchy-feely kind of mom." Because Lola Lily was
always working, my mother was raised by women named Inga
and Nati, domestic workers who were full-time, live-in nannies, cooks, and maids. She remembers Inga fondly, though
she also remembers Inga's husband, a man who made her
and her five sisters uncomfortable because he always seemed
to be watching them. My mother knows what it's like to be
raised by someone other than your mother, and she didn't
want that for my brothers and me.

Nearly fifty years after my parents emigrated, an article
titled "My Family's Slave" was published posthumously by
writer Alex Tizon in the *Atlantic*. Tizon recounts his relationship with a woman he called Lola who, it turns out, was not
a family elder as the name suggests, but, he concludes, an
enslaved person. "She was 18 years old when my grandfather
gave her to my mother as a gift, and when my family moved
to the United States, we brought her with us," Tizon writes.[1]
As I read I wondered if my mother had, on some level years
ago, been aware that she was avoiding a similar situation.
Of not only being responsible for someone else, but someone
who may not have joined her family entirely of their own will.

Having domestic help would no doubt have made my
mom's life easier—she worked outside the home for my entire childhood, long eight-plus-hour days. But my parents
took some satisfaction in "doing it on their own," buying into

the American ethos of individualism, pulling themselves up by their bootstraps. It made for long hours, sore bodies, and a sometimes lonely life, but that was their American Dream.

WHENEVER WE WENT BACK TO the Philippines, adjusting to having domestic help was strange: someone scurrying to cook breakfast as soon as we were up, telling us to leave our dishes on the table, retrieving dirty clothes from our room at some unknown and undetected time, and then leaving them washed and neatly folded on the edge of our beds. As a kid, I was confused by their roles in the households, how I was supposed to interact with them, especially since there was a language barrier. As I got older, I felt more uncomfortable: I had been raised to clear my plate, wash dishes, to separate whites from colors, to put away my laundry. "I'm not your maid," my mother would tell us. But in the Philippines, there was always a maid, and Ima, who intimidated me, would bark at us to let them do their work. At first, I saw the relationship as only one of power and subservience, but life has complicated that impression.

Over time, I saw my mother begin to defer to the domestic workers' authority. It's their job, she told me later, and refusing to let them do it, however well-intentioned, felt insulting and disrespectful. "Who am I to say I can do their job better than them?" she wondered aloud. "I can't!" My mother stays out of their way now, but she always brings gifts for each woman in her balikbayan boxes—usually Victoria's Secret lotions and body sprays—and I'm pretty sure she slips them cash at the end of every trip, just as we're about to leave for the airport.

At Ima's house, Ate Nancy was in charge of the kitchen for many years. When I crave bulalo, tinola, and munggo, it's Ate Nancy's versions that I want. Eventually, Nancy left Ima's house and set up a canteen restaurant adjacent to the supermarket. She's still very much a part of the scene—she'll show up in the kitchen to supervise cooks, and we hired her to babysit our younger daughter when we went out one night.

Ate Celia has worked for my Tita Ginny for nearly fifty years. She's been there for the births of three of my cousins, all of whom are in their forties now. Celia was there through the sudden death of the family patriarch, Tito Albert, and all the grief that still penetrates the family. I believe she is loved dearly. I love her. She is small but so physically strong, which manifests in the sturdiest, most comforting hug. The first time I came back to the Philippines with my older daughter, I couldn't wait to introduce her to Celia, who immediately picked her up to play with her. On another trip, when Noli was a toddler, she wore a turquoise gingham blouse, the straps of which kept falling off her shoulders. Unbeknownst to me, Celia found the blouse and shortened the straps, hand-sewing them. I was touched and grateful, but I also wasn't sure how to feel—had she done it out of love or a sense of obligation?

I want to ask Celia if we feel the same affection for each other, but I don't have the language, and for that I feel stupid and ashamed. But it's not simply a language barrier that stands in our way. Even if I did speak fluent Tagalog, how do you speak across a power differential? Is it possible to ever get to the truth of the relationship?

I'm not entirely comfortable with household help as I see it in the Philippines—the potential for abuse is high, and the tone in which people speak to domestic workers rubs me the wrong way. But it does strike me as a more honest way of living. On Mother's Day a few years ago, my cousin Peng composed a thoughtful Instagram post with pictures of her family's yaya, saying she would never be able to raise her three kids without her.

In the United States domestic work is defined by its invisibility, treated as an afterthought. It's marked by shame, a shame my mother rejected when she chose not to bring a domestic worker with her to America. It's also marked by people's sense of entitlement, that they deserve access to this cheap, essential labor. There is the expectation that the Black and brown women doing this work should stay hidden to keep the system running smoothly. Typically, these women don't appear in photos with the children they care for because they are the ones taking the pictures of the families, or because they are busy doing something else entirely.

ACCORDING TO OXFAM, IF WOMEN around the world made minimum wage for all the unpaid hours of care work they performed in 2019, they would have earned $10.9 trillion. In America alone, they would have earned $1.5 trillion.[2] Because care work remains unpaid, these astounding numbers do not factor into gross domestic product or economic growth.

How did we get to this place where essential work is so devalued? Two crucial lenses to view care work through are capitalism, the system in which trade and industry are privatized and controlled by owners for profit, and colonization, the action of taking control of the land and Indigenous people of an area. At the heart of both lies the impulse to draw a distinct line between beings with power and beings to be dominated, to create cultural binaries of civilized versus natural, modern versus primitive, with what is supposedly civilized and modern being superior.

"The rise of capitalism gave us the idea . . . that most women, Indigenous peoples, slaves, and colonized people everywhere were not fully human and thus not full members of society," write Patel and Moore. "These were people who were not—or were only barely—human."[3] Classifying a huge swath of the population in this way allowed their lives and labor to be cheapened.

Reproductive labor is all the work needed to sustain a productive workforce for generations. It includes caring for children, adults, and the elderly; household chores; and keeping everyone in the household emotionally and physically healthy. Reproductive labor can be performed by mothers, other family members, or hired workers. The common denominator is that the work is either unpaid or low-wage. Many classify the work as unskilled, a myth used to perpetuate a class system that designates some people as less worthy than others.

The association of caregiving with women and the domestic sphere, versus "real work" with men, money, and activities outside the home, runs deep. But these are fairly recent concepts, historically speaking. "The division between 'home' and 'workplace' didn't exist in feudal Europe [where] women worked as doctors, butchers, teachers, retailers, and smiths," writes labor journalist Sarah Jaffe. "Under capitalism, though . . . their work was defined as a natural resource, laying outside the sphere of market relations."[4]

Placing reproductive labor outside the capitalist sphere is what upholds the entire system. Mothers and caregivers participate in the arrangement, by force if necessary. If those who do "professional" work had to commensurately pay the care workers who made their work possible, there would be less profit to be made. Without us, the system falls apart.

The work of mothering—reproductive labor—remains out of sight and out of mind to many because it occurs in the home. This private, domestic space is deemed the domain of women and the extent of our political and social power is expected to be exercised there: household managers, volunteer PTA members. Patel and Moore call this confinement of women, which began in the seventeenth century, the "Great Domestication."

Domestication moved people away from communal living and removed the social and connective aspects of all labor. Men ventured out and worked for employers, in fields and factories, and earned an individual wage. Women stayed in and oversaw the home, where they kept men fed and comfortable, and gave birth to the next generation of workers. This paved the way for the promotion of the nuclear family as the primary way to organize our lives: a single household unit with private property (a wife was property), where the children she raised became the way to protect and pass down wealth. This arrangement cemented the notion that domestic work is women's work, natural and good, done with no expectation of compensation: a labor of love. The modern neoliberal nuclear family, with its ethos of each household going it alone, prevails today.

After the Great Depression, which left so many Americans destitute, the federal government stepped in to help families. To that end, the New Deal established an American Family wage, a guaranteed minimum wage that would be enough to support a working husband, a housewife, and a couple of children. That grand idea was doomed in predictably American ways: lawmakers from the South didn't believe Black men and women should be entitled to the same wages and opportunities as white people. So, the protections excluded two types of laborers: agricultural workers, who were mainly Black men, and domestic workers, the majority of whom were Black women.

Little progress has been made toward fair pay for domestic work. The division between home and work remains paramount to the system we live under. Most people still agree that you toil at work, then come home to be cared for (mostly by women). Since the 1960s, when women's liberation encouraged women to find meaning and power in their lives by pursuing work outside the home, their participation in the waged workforce has steadily risen. But as Jaffe notes, in the current age when many women work both outside and inside of the home, "We hear a lot about 'work-life' balance, but not enough about how, for everyone, 'life' (code for 'family') means 'unpaid work.'"[5]

In the midst of the pandemic, at an emotional low, I entered the hours I spent tending to my family and our home into an online Invisible Labor Calculator to see how much my work might be worth.[6] It was created by journalist Amy Westervelt, who used Bureau of Labor Statistics data to assign an hourly wage to different tasks—washing dishes, considering the emotional needs of family members, doing yard work, cooking, etc. I was floored when the calculator told me my annual wage should be over $300,000, which would make being a domestic worker the highest-paying job I've ever had. By far.

"BEHIND EVERY OFFICE OR MINE there is the hidden work of millions of women who have consumed their life, their labor, producing the labor power that works in those factories, schools, offices, and mines,"[7] writes Silvia Federici.

When most of us imagine economies, domestic or international, we picture workers toiling in factories or offices, money being wire transferred, stocks and bonds traded: all activities that play out in public, covered by the media, highly visible. But the global economy is driven just as much by domestic labor—happening in laundry rooms, nurseries, performed on hands and knees, sponge or toilet brush in hand. Free and commodified care work not only makes formal economies possible, it drives international migration and the transfer of millions of dollars across borders and continents. The global economy is driven as much by care as so-called productive labor.

"White class-privileged women in the United States have historically freed themselves of reproductive labor by purchasing the low-wage services of women of color," writes Rhacel Salazar Parreñas in her study of Filipina immigration and international reproductive labor.[8]

Filipinx people are employed as nannies, house cleaners, and elder-care workers in over 130 countries throughout Asia, the Middle East, Europe, and the United States. The middle- and upper-class American women who employ them are primarily white.

I'm Pinay, my husband is white, and we have relied on my mother's unpaid labor, as well as the paid labor of immigrants and Latina, Black, and Chinese women to care for our children. I continue to navigate my place as an American woman of color who is financially privileged. I've been mistaken by strangers for my light-skinned daughters' caretaker, which has angered me and also forced me to question why it makes me angry. This tension has made me bold, willing to speak out in solidarity with caregivers in some instances. At other times, it's made me quiet and embarrassed. I can claim otherness, I know it intimately, but I have always known that, if things fall apart, I could ask for help, that I would never be left destitute or totally alone.

We like to tell ourselves that American women are better off—"freer"—than other women around the world, in part because we can easily work outside the home. But we are not free or unburdened from other people. We are dependent on our nannies, cleaners, personal Instacart shoppers, Door Dash delivery drivers, parents, co-parents, chosen family, and in-laws. The domestic load is as heavy as ever, but if we have the means, we spread it out among multiple people. This is not real progress. White women's reliance on the low-wage labor of women of color actually deepens racial inequities in America—and around the world.

"Migrant Filipino domestic workers hire poorer women in the Philippines to perform the reproductive labor that they are performing for wealthier women in receiving nations," writes Salazar Parreñas, who conducted extensive interviews with Filipinx domestic workers in Italy and Los Angeles. (While Latinx women dominate the field of household maintenance in the Los Angeles area and across the United States, migrant Filipinas comprise most of the elder care in the city.[9]) She calls this arrangement the "international transfer of caretaking."

This international transfer of workers creates a low-wage working class in America, as well as in the Philippines. Pinay women, even those with a high school or college degree, choose to go abroad because domestic worker wages in industrialized nations are still higher than the wages for professional workers in the Philippines. Salazar Parreñas calculates that Filipina migrant workers might make around $1,700 a month abroad, while their monthly salary at home would be less than $200.[10]

While many Filipinos would prefer to stay home, closer to their children, friends, and extended families, it makes better economic sense to leave. Their predicament reminds me of a slogan on a Wages for Housework flyer from the 1970s: a fist holding a bundle of cash pushing forcefully through the center of the women's symbol: "We can't afford to work for love."

IN THE TWENTIETH CENTURY, ONE of the most notable efforts to improve the lives of care workers and mothers was led by the National Welfare Rights Organization (NWRO). Established in 1966 and led by Black women such as Johnnie Tillmon, the NWRO organized for expanded access and entitlements for women eligible for welfare, which at the time was called Aid to Families with Dependent Children (AFDC). Because white government officials wanted to regulate who received these benefits and worried that poor, "undeserving" women would take advantage of the program, AFDC recipients were surveilled and subject to home inspections. The NWRO used direct action—holding sit-ins and disrupting welfare offices—as well as marches and rallies to lobby for greater benefits and the elimination of punitive policy elements. Eventually the NWRO started a campaign to benefit all people in America, not just AFDC mothers and families.

In a 1972 article for *Ms.* magazine titled "Welfare Is a Women's Issue," Tillmon laid out their vision for a Guaranteed Adequate Income:

> There would be no "categories"—men, women, children, single, married, kids, no kids—just poor people who need aid. You'd get paid according to need and

family size only and that would be upped as the cost of living goes up.

In other words, I'd start paying women a living wage for doing the work we are already doing—child-raising and house-keeping. And the welfare crisis would be over, just like that.[11]

The NWRO came very close to winning a guaranteed income policy. President Richard Nixon, of all people, put forth a Family Assistance Plan that would have given a basic income to more than ten million people. Ultimately, Nixon's plan did not pass and instead America got Ronald Reagan and the racist 1980s narrative of the "welfare queen." But that the NWRO came as close as it did to enacting a guaranteed income for caregivers should give us hope that it is possible. Though they did not succeed in everything they fought for, the NWRO and its allies did improve conditions for thousands of families, helping them access all the benefits they were legally entitled to. As Tillmon said, "Maybe it is we poor welfare women who will really liberate women in this country."

CARE IS EXPECTED TO BE cheap the world over, in part because the global economy doesn't have the ability to properly value care work; conventional economic measures—concepts such as supply, demand, and markets—fall woefully short. But the failures of imagination that have led to this moment don't have to dictate that care work not be assigned monetary value going forward, or that we shouldn't try. If mothers and care workers were to withhold their labor, whole countries and economies would grind to a halt.

How might we properly value care? It requires a new way of seeing the work and the world, bringing forth a new vision. We need to question our entire system of values. Productivity, efficiency, and hustle must share the stage with wholeness, health, stability, and self-regard. We must start by acknowledging mothering as highly skilled work that deserves respect and compensation.

One of the most important aspects of the NWRO's legacy is its emphasis on the power of collectivity. The intent of their work was not merely to benefit the poorest women they were organizing, but also mothers, housewives, and all people in poverty. By seeing beyond divisions of sex, race, and class, they led with commonality and shared humanity—the solidarity needed to address the cause of all economic inequality. Tillmon wrote that for women on welfare, liberation is "a matter of survival." Their analysis was similar to that of the Combahee River Collective, a group of Black feminists who believed that "when you see all of the issues as being intertwined, you look to the root, to what will wipe out the most of your problems; to what will solve the most and improve conditions for as many people as possible; for everyone." The women of Combahee concluded that "capitalism is the problem."[12]

No woman, regardless of race or class, is safe from the expectation of reproductive labor. Even for the richest white women who are able to outsource all the work—when, say, the support system they have built and hired vanishes amid a devastating years-long global health crisis—the work still falls to them.

In July 2020, four months into America's Covid-19 shutdown, writer Deb Perelman published an op-ed in the *New York Times*, announcing her recent, startling realization that mothers don't matter to the country's economy. "Let me say the quiet part loud: In the Covid-19 economy, you're allowed only a kid or a job," she writes.

It's necessary that women like Perelman learn this fact—and that their anger and frustration be spread widely on national media platforms. We need everyone in this fight. But perhaps more significant is that it took a pandemic and its extreme conditions for Perelman to experience this epiphany.

"Despite our own financial strain, we've continued to pay the nanny who used to help shuttle the kids around while we worked, even though she hasn't worked for us since March," Perelman writes, making her privilege clear. "Even if we asked for her help in home schooling our children this fall, who would do so for her school-age children?"[13]

I remember being a little stunned—both grateful for this piece for bringing further attention to the issue, but also feeling cynical and petty, wondering if Perelman had ever considered her nanny's children before, what daily life was like for that family. As I read the comments on the piece, I was comforted that I wasn't alone.

"Many of us who made our way into the working world during the great recession already felt this long before Covid," someone wrote. "I would suggest that this is a much bigger problem and you are just now noticing it because the pandemic forces inconveniences on people who are not used to dealing with them."

Plenty of white and privileged women are now discovering that all women are characterized by a condition of servitude. That even women who can avoid some or all housework are still beholden to it. That, as Federici writes, "we are all in a servant relation with respect to the entire male world."[14]

Like the NWRO, the Wages for Housework network didn't achieve its ultimate goal of securing payment for work done by women in the home, but it did offer a clear and powerful perspective, as well as important analyses and ideas that we can look to today—particularly, in Federici's words, "that raising children and taking care of people is a social responsibility."

What would happen if those of us who mother insisted that our bodies and our work be fully visible and valued?

We got a glimpse on October 24, 1975, when women in Iceland staged the Iceland Women's Strike. An estimated 90 percent of women did not show up for work that day—in and outside of the home—and it brought Iceland's economy to its knees. Factories, schools, and nurseries were closed, and men either called in to stay home from work or brought their children with them. In the decades that have followed, some of the strike's agenda have taken hold. In 2018 Iceland became the first country in the world to require employers with more than twenty-five employees to give women and men equal pay for equal work.[15] Part of the strike's legacy is showing that it is possible to organize on a mass scale, and that such a show of solidarity made lasting impressions that are still invoked today.[16]

Mothering can no longer be considered supplementary or inferior to wage labor. If we reframe domestic work as essential labor and insist upon its centrality in a global labor movement, we create opportunities for solidarity among caregivers, mothers, and all workers. Unity can exist across gender identities, international borders, and disparate industries, rooted in any work that exploits an invisible labor force. When we insist on the monetary value of mothering, we do nothing less than redefine work. We redraw the image of workers to be more inclusive, to consider people's health and humanity. We proclaim that care, maintenance, and a sustainable pace of life are essential to our labor.

Redefining the workplace, as so many of us have done during the Covid-19 pandemic, advances this vision. Work, we all now know, has never been confined to the office or the field or the factory. It was always happening in the kitchen, garage, and backyard.

Domestic spaces—our hallways, sofas, and dining room tables—are much more than places where families gather. They are where essential workers broker wages and terms of employment, which often have international consequence. As Argentinian theorist and activist Verónica Gago writes, our homes are "spaces of practical internationalism where global care chains are assembled, where reproductive labor is negotiated."[17] We have been trained to view our houses and apartments as private refuges, but they must also be seen for what they are: job sites where millions of dollars of the global economy are directly exchanged.

Those of us who demand respect and recompense for

mothering are, in Federici's words, "seen as nagging bitches, not as workers in struggle."[18] I want to believe that Federici is writing squarely about a past, one we will never return to. Because we are no different from ride share drivers, sanitation workers, welders, teachers, physicians, nurses. We are no different from our nannies and childcare workers and the people cleaning our homes. We share the struggle of domestic workers in the Philippines such as Ate Celia, Ate Perla, Ate Nancy, and Inga. Our issues are the same as the women we have paid to take care of our children—for me, that means I stand with Maria, Josephine, Huang Ping, Belen, Ceci, Mari, Marta, Sandra, and Titi.

It makes white women uncomfortable to think that they are no different from their hired help. What they chase—and have been given—is validation, acceptance, and success, but only on terms set by white men. Proximity to power, however real that feels, is a simpler choice than solidarity. True allyship lives in relationships, true solidarity requires giving up some comfort, material resources, and power—and sharing it with others. To confront your own internalized misogyny and racism is humbling, destabilizing. Can white women do this? Can they acknowledge and own their whiteness and its accompanying entitlement? Can they get past themselves and get on our level?

Only then do we have a chance. In Johnnie Tillmon's words, "No woman can be liberated, until all women get off their knees."[19]

3

MOTHERING AS
EROTIC LABOR

My mother sits in a green vinyl chair next to a blue-and-white faux marble counter scattered with jewelry and glass bottles. At the other end is a shell-shaped sink, the kind a mermaid would have. The air is steamy and sweet, thick with the scent of Jean Naté After Bath Splash, drugstore lotions, and powders. I sit on a little stool at her feet, my head sideways in her lap. With careful, callused fingers she takes the silver pantutule and swirls it around the outer edges of my ear, then works her way in deep, scooping out my soft, crumbly white ear wax. She wipes the wax on a square of toilet paper so I can study it afterward—she knows I love to look at it, sometimes smell it, roll it in my fingers. When she is done with my left ear, I turn and face her stomach. I close my eyes and feel this soft part of her body rise and fall and brush against my face with each breath as she cleans my right ear. There's no distance between us; I inhale her scent, am one with her heat. Even today, I can return to this feeling in an instant.

The ear spoon is a flimsy thing, made of cheap aluminum. In less caring hands, it could cut the delicate skin lining an ear canal or puncture an eardrum. My mother wielded it expertly, tenderly excavating my body's waste. Cleaning my ears right after a bath made it easier—body damp and relaxed, ear wax softened. But I preferred having it done when everything was dry—I liked feeling my mother's effort, her digging and the resistance, the careful vigilance required.

"For the Vietnamese, a lot of love is articulated through service," says the poet Ocean Vuong in an interview I read. "We don't say, I love you. We cook, we massage, we *cạo gió*, we scratch each other's backs."[1] A surge of recognition runs through me.

Sometimes, as a weekend treat, our family had champorado with tuyo for breakfast. I whined about having to separate the fish from the tinik that sometimes stuck in my throat and made me gag. My mom painstakingly pulled the meat from the fine bones to make a pile of salty fish for me to mix into the dark porridge.

My mother certainly told my brothers and me that she loved us, but always in English, not her native language. When she immigrated to the United States she became fluent in English and much of American culture. But I sense that she might still be more comfortable giving and receiving love in demonstrative ways. Like so many immigrants, she adapted but can never abandon what was instilled in her body.

For much of my life, I thought words were the most

important form of expression, but I don't think that way now. The body conveys love so much more eloquently. Hearing "I love you" is nothing compared to feeling it, your body absorbing the message from another. Before we learn verbal language, we communicate through our bodies. The only way a young child can comprehend love is physically.

HAVING A BODY IS GENERALLY treated as an inconvenience, especially a body that has constant, evolving needs. The racism, colorism, homophobia, transphobia, sexism, and ableism that define American culture insist, in both small and big ways, that those of us who differ from the perceived norm might be better off without our bodies. Having our basic physical needs met—the foundation for being able to freely pursue what we please—is a human right. It's not a privilege bestowed on us through working or proving our deservedness; we are born deserving. We feed and tend to a baby without question, even through the haze of sleep deprivation and exhaustion. There is no reason that generosity should vanish as we age.

I reject the American idea of "earning a living." I am alive and I don't need to do anything to earn my existence. We don't have to prove that we are worthy of comfort, ease, pleasure, or satisfaction. I don't need a job to contribute something to my community—I just need to be me. Mothering shows children that there is nothing wrong with having a body and having needs. More important, it establishes the expectation that having those needs met is essential, a minimum guarantee in this life.

Audre Lorde terms this vital, physical energy the erotic. "We tend to think of the erotic as an easy, tantalizing sexual arousal," she writes. "I speak of the erotic as the deepest life force, a force which moves us toward living in a fundamental way."[2]

Mothering is sensual—endemic to the body and bringing both profound joy and fulfillment. It cultivates and nurtures a child's life force and essence. It is labor that can bestow a primal sense of satisfaction to children and caregivers alike.

BECAUSE OF THEIR WORK, my parents never shied away from talking about bodies. I knew words such as *autopsy, surgical biopsy, necrosis, frozen section, carcinoma, catheter,* and *rigor mortis* before I was out of elementary school. When I had a dark purple bruise or a hot, swollen mosquito bite, words like *hematoma* and *cellulitis* were tossed out casually. My older brother had severe asthma and eczema as a child, as well as a seafood allergy, so we were all familiar with inhalers, nebulizers, steroids, anaphylaxis. Everyone in both my parents' extended families called my dad for opinions or second opinions about their thyroid, diabetes, high blood pressure, or other diagnoses.

I loved hearing about all the bodies in our lives and what was going on with them. I liked playing with my dad's stethoscope, trying to hear the sound my own body made on the inside, and peeking into my mother's bag of syringes and blue bed pads. For all the talk of body parts and functions, though, we never spoke about being human animals inhabiting our fleshy, organ-filled bodies. We never talked about what it felt like to live, play, and move through the world in them. And we certainly never spoke of the pleasure of being in a body, the pleasure we could give ourselves or others.

My parents' framing of bodies was always clinical. I can't remember a time when I didn't know what a C-section was. I knew my mother had three of them because she was born with a congenital condition: vaginal and uterine septums, her reproductive organs divided in two. C-sections seemed common to me, much more so than the idea of pushing a baby out of my "pekadoodee," which is what my mother called my vagina. (Penises were called "titis.") I also knew my mom didn't know about her vaginal septum until she was pregnant.

I had questions about how she found it, if sex—which she had for the first time on her wedding night—was painful, but I didn't dare ask. I still have questions, but within my family there are some subjects that remain too far out of a comfort zone to properly address. Some things remain unknown.

FOR THE EARLY YEARS OF a child's life, the geography of mothering, more than the house or playground, is the body. No one knows our bodies, or the bodies that we wipe and caress every day, better than ourselves. During pregnancy and throughout the early years of mothering, we are actively discouraged from trusting our instincts by guidebooks and so-called experts.

"As women," Lorde writes, "we have come to distrust that power which rises from our deepest and nonrational knowledge."[3] This keeps us uncertain, small, and afraid. While parenting books mostly leave me agitated, I can't shake something written in 1946 by Dr. Benjamin Spock, a clarion call that cuts through so much noise: "Trust yourself. You know more than you think you do."

Having children has taught me that love is an action verb. And one that can only be performed with our hands and arms and brain and torsos, however imperfect or tired or ungovernable they are. Mothering is acts of service and attention to the body. Drool wiping, hand washing, nose blowing, food spooning, hair brushing, bathing, picking up, pinning down to put clothes on, changing diapers. You move, but you also have to be still. To let them lie on you, to stroke their hair, to study and memorize them.

You simply can't convey with words your dedication to a child. (Arguably, you can't do it with just words with adults either—action is best, but you have a better chance of conveying it in a way that can be intellectually comprehended.) You have to show children with physical attention and affection. And you have to show them over and over and over again.

It is draining, tedious, and repetitive, but the work keeps us close to one another, returns us, again and again, to our own corporeal forms. Physical labor exhausts me, but it makes me more tender. More empathetic, more sensate, more porous. In touch with all the emotions. As Lorde writes, "Erotic is not only a question of what we do; it is a question of how acutely and fully we can feel in the doing."[4]

When my toddler refuses to get dressed or wear anything other than a star dress that is in the washing machine, things can go south quickly. I point out that she has so many clothes, she says she hates them all. I threaten to throw everything away, she dares me to do it. I yell, she yells, I yell and leave the room and she cries, or I just yell and stay put and we stare at each other in a huffy standoff. But sometimes I catch myself before the yelling cycle kicks in. Sometimes I remember I can do something else. Sometimes I take a deep breath. I sit on the floor. I get close, I talk softly. I slow it all down and take another breath, feel my nervous system begin to calm down. Hers does too. I offer a hug, we embrace, we start over. I only succeed at doing this maybe half the time. But when I take a minute, step away, be in the breath, my instinct tells me to stick with it, to stay in it with her, to show her that no matter how angry I am, no matter what she does, no matter how far we push ourselves away from each other, my love for her will always be close, a constant.

A FRIEND OF MINE WORKS at a large social media company. I met her at her office for lunch, where I was overwhelmed by the choices: the salad bar (which gets tossed manually in a bowl by a young Black woman), the stir-fry area, the carved meat station, the smoothie bar. We sat outside on a deck overlooking one of Seattle's sparkling lakes. We talked about the perks of working there, including that she could bring clothes in to be dry-cleaned. You can bring your laundry in too, which she said a fair number of her coworkers did. But she couldn't bring herself to do that—it's just a step too far for me, she explained. As we walked out, at her encouragement, I filled my bag with pamplemousse LaCroix, Pirate's Booty, Kettle chips, and some Justin's dark chocolate peanut butter cups.

There is a joke, not a very good one, that the ultimate goal of companies like this and apps—ones that will come and pick you up and drive you wherever you want, take your food order, let you know when a cook begins making your food, and then give you updates as a driver brings it to your door, the ones that pair you with a stylist to help you pick out clothes—is to replace "your mom." To remove direct physicality from the equation. Indulging in these conveniences is a nice way to give yourself a break, but relying on them deprives you of the satisfaction of knowing and loving yourself enough to tend to your body. It's not shameful to be a fleshy mass, to have needs. It's not inconvenient. It just is.

There is nothing like a body willing to do the work, to lend energy and time, its physical magnificence. And when that work is demanding and done day in and day out, as mothering is, it becomes a commitment that can be felt wholly by a child, a security that they will carry through life. They are worthy and they are safe, and they should never feel anything less than that.

I can touch this feeling, given to me by my own mother, every time my girls put their heads in my lap and I turn my headlamp on, excavating orange fudgy wax from their ears. No bit of them is too much, too smelly or gross—I made every inch of them and I will love and tend to all of them.

THE PANDEMIC REFRACTED OUR LIVES like a prism, bending and distorting the image we have of ourselves, directing light and color into the dark corners of our accepted ways of existing. During this long, strange season many people began to see—for the first time or anew—that what mothers and other caregivers do is highly skilled work.

Our economic system is based on the specious notion that people in the home performing reproductive labor are doing something less valuable than people who go out into the world—into the office or public spaces. "Stay-at-home mom" has long been considered an almost derogatory term, as though the home was somehow maintaining itself.

When you're home all day, toys and mess and clutter accumulate and must be dealt with. The dried fecal matter clinging to the toilet bowl, the slow drain of the bathroom sink, and the soap scum in the bathtub can be ignored only for so long before it starts to seem unhygienic and menacing. Also, we need to change the bedsheets wet with urine, the last frontier of potty training. Someone's gotta get down on their hands and knees to pick up the desiccated pieces of corn and ground beef beneath the dining room table. It's time to vacuum, to get the food bits we cannot see, the dried leaves and dirt tracked in on the bottom of shoes. The barely touched green bean casserole gets scraped into the compost bin, which is about to overflow and needs to be taken out—along with the trash and recycling—on Tuesday. The toddler needs to be reminded of how to wipe properly; there have been skid marks in every pair of underwear this week.

For the body, female or male, neither or both, there is no

getting around the work of keeping yourself alive. Of all the things we take for granted in life, the constant work of the body—giving you the power to breathe without thinking, react to threatening situations, move from one room to the next, digest your food—is one of the most glaring. A healthy, functioning body is always working—multiple systems in tandem, correcting temperature, clearing waste. This is the tremendous work of homeostasis, or balance, and it's not a static state of being. It is dynamic, requiring energy and effort even when we don't realize it.

Childcare and domestic work are maintenance. Fluids, vomit, and mucus abound, the by-products of a being staying alive. We see maintenance work as undesirable, someone else's job to deal with, not worth our precious time. We think progress is outsourcing care and maintenance, further distancing ourselves from it, never adequately compensating the people who do this work. We are deluding ourselves.

SINCE 1968, THE ARTIST Mierle Laderman Ukeles has been exploring the way our culture devalues maintenance work. Ukeles was called to this subject after becoming a mother.

"I was so powerful, giving life and keeping life alive, learning the hum of getting from one breath to the next, and learning the mind-bending boredom of repetitive task work," she says. "I felt like two people in the same body. The free artist and the mother maintenance worker. I never worked so hard in my life trying to keep everything together."[5]

In 1969 Ukeles wrote "Manifesto for Maintenance Art,"

a proposal for an exhibition titled "CARE." In it Ukeles set forth a plan to live in a museum with her husband and child, doing the work she would do around their home including sweeping the floors, dusting, and cooking. Ukeles connected the reproductive labor of mothering to the professional maintenance jobs of janitors and sanitation workers:

> Maintenance is a drag; it takes all the fucking time . . .
> The culture confers lousy status on maintenance jobs =
> Minimum wages, housewives = no pay[6]

While studying a document from the New York City planning department, Ukeles noticed that work was divided into two categories, Development and Maintenance. Development was linear progress, advancement, and "individual creation." Maintenance, on the other hand, was circular and repetitive: "keep the dust off the pure individual creation; preserve the new; sustain the change; protect progress." Development, she noted, was associated with maleness, maintenance with the female.

Ukeles accepted a position as artist-in-residence at the New York City Department of Sanitation in 1977, a post she still holds today. As part of her tenure she developed a work of art, conducted from 1979 to 1980, called "Touch Sanitation Performance." Ukeles spent eleven months meeting over 8,500 individual department employees in person. She visited sanitation crews, shadowed them as they performed their duties, interviewed them, and took the time to understand the particulars of their work. She pulled sixteen-hour shifts. After every conversation with a sanitation worker, she shook each of their hands and said, "Thank you for keeping New York City alive."[7]

Those who mother are the sanitation workers of bodies—handling the refuse, the filth and putrescence, living in the stink. Ukeles's art shows that what garbage handlers and caregivers do is nothing less than what keeps us alive.

In 2020, as Covid-19 shut down New York City, Ukeles and the Queens Museum revived "Touch Sanitation" to acknowledge the city's essential workers. Sanitation and transit employees never stopped working, even as countless buildings went dark around them; the workers put themselves at great risk to keep the city's infrastructure running. The new exhibit, called "For → Forever," was a three-part display of public art at prominent locations: a billboard in Times Square, the outside of the Queens Museum, and over two thousand digital displays throughout the MTA subway and rail systems. Ukeles chose to use a color palette of safety green and emergency orange, the same colors in the uniforms of maintenance workers. The colors, she said, signify that "the person inside here is precious." Each day, essential workers could see this message while they were working or commuting:

> Dear Service Worker,
>   "Thank you for keeping NYC alive!"
> For → forever . . .

It's both remarkable—and damning—that Ukeles's message, unchanged over forty years, is as timely and relevant as ever. In her own words, "The manifesto is a world vision and a call for revolution for the workers of maintenance, these are the workers of survival."[8]

As part of her original "CARE" proposal, Ukeles planned to ask fifty people—"50 different classes and kinds" including maids, construction workers, nurses, doctors, teachers, children, criminals, and movie stars—about their relationship to maintenance. Her proposed questions were:

- What you think maintenance is;
- How you feel about spending whatever parts of your life you spend on maintenance activities;
- What is the relationship between maintenance and freedom;
- What is the relationship between maintenance and life's dreams.[9]

The last two stuck with me for months after I first read them. Turning them over and over in my mind, I thought about how, when our health and safety are maintained, either by ourselves or others, we have the freedom to pursue our dreams. And it is clear to me that our freedom and dreams should never come at the cost of someone else's. I was curious what my mother—the person who maintained my body for so long—would have to say about Ukeles's questions. She was a little nervous when we started and veered off-topic, but when I let her talk instead of trying to lead her back to the questions, she opened up:

Everything is maintenance! Even your body needs maintenance, oh my gosh. Even my hair needs maintenance. Once you let go of things, it's harder to keep up with it. I think everybody has their own priorities in life and I place a high priority on maintenance and cleanliness.

You know the story of Mary Magdalene, who washed the feet of Jesus and dried them with her hair? I'm like her sister, Martha, the one who was so busy around the house and said, "Jesus, why don't you stop talking and let Mary help me clean up?" Well, I'm Martha, I'll do the dishes.[10] I've always been like this.

Anyway maintenance, really it's the core. It's everything.

WHETHER A COMMITMENT TO MAINTENANCE is part of our nature, an obligation we begrudgingly fill, or something that brings us genuine joy, there is no getting around it. The poet Marge Piercy writes that, "The work of the world is as common as mud. / Botched, it smears the hands, crumbles to dust. / But the thing worth doing well done / has a shape that satisfies, clean and evident. . . . The pitcher cries for water to carry / And a person for work that is real."[11]

Ever since I read that poem in high school I've wondered what "real work" is, and sensed that my understanding of it was out of step with the world. I never really wanted to be a professional; all I knew was that I wanted whatever I did to matter. I believe writing matters, of course, but nothing has ever felt more real to me than the work of caring. That energy and effort to maintain—ourselves, our loved ones, our community—has always felt substantial, true, visceral, and, yes, real to me. I don't believe care work has to wreck us. This labor can be shared, social, collective—and transformative.

In 1881, 98 percent of Black women in the city of Atlanta were domestic workers, and the majority of the women worked as laundresses, washing and ironing the clothes of wealthy white women. Before the widespread use of washing machines and dryers, laundry was hard labor. The women carried gallons of water from wells and pumps, set them to boil, then washed clothes and linens with soap they made themselves. After drying the laundry, they'd iron it using heavy tools.

"I could clean my hearth good and nice and set my irons in front of the fire and iron all day [with]out stopping. . . . I cooked and ironed at the same time," said laundress Sarah Hill.[12]

One benefit of the work was that it could be done in a group, with other women in the neighborhood, outside if the weather was nice. As they washed, they could talk, sharing difficulties, stories, and complaints about their employers. They built solidarity. In July 1881, twenty laundresses formed the Washing Society, and began organizing for more respect, autonomy, and a set wage. To achieve this, they planned to strike. In just three weeks, the Society grew from twenty to three thousand members. The laundresses succeeded.[13]

One hundred years later, in her 1981 book *Women, Race and Class,* Angela Davis argued that housework should no longer be private. She envisioned the industrialization of housework: "teams of trained and well-paid workers, moving from dwelling to dwelling, engineering technologically advanced cleaning machinery." She insisted that this service be accessible and affordable to working-class people. Davis also believed that childcare and meal preparation should be socialized, something done together, rather than alone in our individual homes.[14]

There is no reason maintenance work should be hidden, no reason it should happen in isolation. By nature it is social, and the shared connection that happens when we put our bodies to work together stays in our bodies, mixed with the camaraderie we feel with others. It is the erotic that Lorde speaks of, rooted in the fundamentals of our existence, fueling the animating forces of our life.

The physical closeness that my mother missed out on receiving from her own mother was given freely and generously to me. Even though she worked full-time and couldn't be with me every time I needed her, I still remember the care, the intimacy, the tending. To this day my body knows the feeling of being held. We give the people we mother our bodies, and what they will recall is our presence and heat, the animal closeness. Before and after words come, this is what we need—this connectedness—the last thing we find ourselves groping for at night when quiet descends and we are alone with our soft selves in need of comfort.

4

MOTHERING AS HUMAN INTERDEPENDENCE

The texture of my childhood is brown, plush, and abundant. Upholstered bucket seats and a backseat that unfolded into a bed three kids could lie down on. Our family logged seemingly endless hours and miles in our van, a living room on wheels: carpeted, with blinds and a removable faux-wood drink holder, even a little nook under the backseat for me to read or sleep. My brother Jay and I climbed the ladder on its back to stunt for family photos on the roof. I ate so many Filet-O-Fish sandwiches and Chicken McNuggets with hot mustard sauce en route to Buffalo; New York City; or Scarsdale, New York, to visit my dad's brother Uncle Ging and his wife, Aunt Kathy, or my mom's sister Tita Fe and my cousin Ate Bonnie, or another of my mom's five sisters, Tita Ginny. She and her husband, Tito Albert, had five kids, and the youngest, Len Len, was my favorite cousin. Technically she was my Ate, but only by three months. Her family lived in the Philippines but spent a few years in the States in the 1980s, during which we saw them as often as possible.

At Thanksgiving and Christmas tables overflowing with turkey and mashed potatoes, but also chicken embutido, siopao, and bibingka, we'd be joined by various family members who flew in from Canada and California: Lola Lily, the family matriarch; Tita Nene, an inscrutable older sister who almost became a nun and now lived in the same building as Lola; Tita Tessie, my ninang and fellow bunso, a "free spirit" from Berkeley and her daughters Monique and Danielle. If we were lucky, the oldest Zaragoza sister, Tita Baby, and her husband, Tito Pons, along with one or more of their four kids, would make the trip from West Covina.

I had a particular affection for Tita Baby—I loved her smile and soft skin and saw myself in her round face—and her only daughter, my Ate Dally, because their family had briefly lived with ours when they first immigrated to America. At the time I was just two years old, while Tita Baby's kids were high schoolers. Always laughing, they'd tell the same story over and over—how I had invented my own word, *abukaniya*, which I'd use to express delight or anger, depending on my toddler mood, with exaggerated body language, facial expressions, and tone. That, as a child, I created a private language for my emotions feels core to who I am. I'm grateful to them for this memory I could never have on my own.

Holidays and summer vacations and impromptu weekends were joyous and cacophonous; I have no idea what the adults did all that time, and I didn't care. I passed the hours playing Spit, jumping rope, making stop-motion animation videos with toys and clay figures, defending myself from the torment of my kuyas, doing karaoke on the Minus One machine. We cousins ran feral and free until mealtime, when we'd all come together and the titos would drink beer and tease us and the titas would set the table and make tsismis. Ate Celia was always there, too, corralling kids, laughing her loud easy laugh, washing the dishes. Nighttime was a big slumber party, three or six of us girls squeezed into one room; sometimes I'd wake to go pee in the night and find Len Len sleepwalking through the dark hallways in her yellow nightgown. At the end of each trip, I'd crawl reluctantly back into the van, heavier now thanks to a cooler filled with leftovers, and we'd make our way home. Those drives were as silent as the white lines of the highway.

Our house in Pennsylvania was comfortable and spacious, but quiet. I'd take the bus home after school and walk the half mile down our gravel road to an empty house. We were latchkey kids, and my brothers had little interest in playing with me, so I'd walk in our backyard woods and lie down on a large patch of moss that I thought of as my own personal rug to look up at the tall hemlocks and daydream. Inside, *Kate & Allie, You Can't Do That on Television,* and *Growing Pains* were my companions. One or both of my parents were always home in time to make dinner, and it was important to them that we sit down together every night to Filipino food if they had time, or Hamburger Helper if they didn't. I had friends, of course, but we lived "out in the country," not in town or

close to any of them. My parents had friends too: Mrs. Alber-
tini, Mrs. Miller, Mrs. Kennedy, Mr. and Mrs. Nugent. There
were just a few folks—Sam and Linda, Uncle Paul and Aunt
Mary—whom I could call by familiar names. Our lives were
full, but when I think about daily life, I remember a lot of
lonely hours. I wonder if my parents felt the same way, another question I'm afraid to ask.

I viewed community as something that we lacked, though
I know that's not entirely true. I wanted to live somewhere
else—maybe Berkeley, where my Filipina-Belgian cousins
had friends named Aram who were Jewish; or New York City,
where there was an entire neighborhood of Asian people and
dim sum and I might have a chance to be cool like the editors
of *Sassy* magazine. I dreamed of West Covina, Daly City, or
Stockton—hometown of Dawn Bohulano Mabalon, the Filipina teenage editor in chief of *Sassy's* 1991 reader-produced
issue. I dreamed of living anyplace with large Filipino communities, with Philippine grocery stores, or just a Jollibee or
a Goldilocks Bakery. What, I wondered, would I be like if I
was from Milpitas? If I felt on some level that I actually be-
longed, wasn't aware at every moment that I was somehow
different. And, I wondered: What would my parents be like
if they could speak their first languages, Tagalog and Kapampangan, every day? If they could buy ampalaya leaves and ma-
capuno ice cream at the supermarket and run into friends
while shopping?

We all turned out fine. Not unscathed, but fine. My parents loved us wholly and generously. But they were focused
on survival, fitting in, and so, it seemed to me, were my

brothers. While I was slurping sinigang and spitting out pork neck bones, my brother Jay wanted Roman Meal bread with Smucker's Goober Grape spread. Neither he nor our oldest brother, Pete, seemed keen to join my dad on his yearly visits back to the Philippines, where he would visit his parents and drink San Miguel beer with his brothers while I played with dozens of cousins each day, buying sodas in plastic bags from street vendors, skin polka-dotted red with mosquito bites, and developing a deep tan.

No, it was only me who was plagued by noticing the differences, who always wondered if people were making fun of my parents or our family, who knew there was no hope of ever fitting in, not really, and resenting our little town, wanting more. I'm still haunted by my best friend Lisa's senior yearbook quote, from Solzhenitsyn, whom I'd never even heard of (Lisa was one of the only Black students in our school and the valedictorian): "Sometimes I feel quite distinctly that what is inside me is not all of me. There is something else, quite lofty, some fragment of the world spirit. Don't you feel that?"

God, yes.

Where we lived—the people we lived among—never felt like enough to me. But for my parents it seemed to suffice. After all, they had come such a long way, endured so much to settle in this town and create a stable foundation for us. Maybe this had to be the place. This little rural borough was going to be home, they would make it work, even if that meant doing it mostly on their own.

2021. I ASK MY PARENTS what they think life would be like for them if they had never left the Philippines. As soon as the words fly from my lips, cartoon butterflies, I want to grab them and stuff them back in because, really, what's the point? What's done is done. What could I possibly hear that would be helpful?

"I was already going, no matter what," my mother replies. And that is that.

"She was already going when we met," my father says. "If we didn't get married, and I didn't go with her? I would have just married someone else. Then I'd probably be a struggling doctor in the provinces . . . and actually I'd probably be sick or dead with Covid right now. How's that?"

This is the immigrant practicality I love most, and am equally infuriated by, in them. The subtext being: What the fuck kind of pointless question is this?

Of course I have some guesses. Many of my cousins, my age and even older, still live with their parents, or lived with them well into their twenties or thirties, after they'd started families of their own. Intergenerational homes are the norm; living together for many years is simply how family operates—unlike in the United States, being independent isn't necessarily a goal.

Central to precolonial Philippine culture is bayanihan, which means communal solidarity. Its roots lie in the shared labor of farming, child-rearing, house-building, and house-moving. Throughout Philippine folk art, you'll find a recurring image of a group of people moving a nipa hut hoisted on bamboo sticks, à la Cleopatra being carried on a litter. In a tropical, monsoon-heavy climate, flooding is not uncommon. Through bayanihan, a community could relocate a family by lifting the home and moving it to higher ground.

Bayanihan, according to historian Luis H. Francia, was the cornerstone of Indigenous Filipino communities known as barangays. In this social context, "producers owned their means of production, and any surplus from a bountiful harvest was stored against a rainy day or for barter . . . In a word, the archipelagic barangay was not only precolonial but also precapitalist."[1]

Francia cites the Banaue rice terraces (which many Filipinos like me were raised to proudly call the "eighth wonder of the world") built by the Ifugao people of Northern Luzon as an enduring example of bayanihan. Carved out of the rock of the Cordillera Mountains at treacherous heights and angles, the terraces, which are still in use today, required tremendous coordination and effort to build. "Organizing the labor, building up the paddies, and devising the placement of rocks and irrigation canals were daunting challenges that required a tight, cohesive, and efficient social structure," he writes.[2]

In modern American culture, that sort of tight-knit community structure seems increasingly rare. For centuries, extended personal networks have been eroded, replaced with privatized jobs and small, isolated kin units. "The extended family and relationships that could sustain families were transformed and professionalized," write Patel and Moore.[3] A lack of shared responsibility and interconnectedness makes it difficult to find solutions for needs more easily addressed in

community, such as childcare, meal preparation, and household maintenance. It leads to isolation and an every-family-
for-themselves mentality. It leaves parents feeling common
domestic strains as personal problems rather than struc-
tural ones.

"Neoliberal family life has turned the very idea of account-
ability to others into a dreadful burden," writes sociologist
Kathryn Jezer-Morton. "If you're looking to optimize your
schedule for maximum efficiency, having to pause and account for someone else's pace and needs—someone who isn't
even related to you!—throws a spanner in the works."[4]

I'm not trying to romanticize or fetishize the past, but the
simple fact is that for centuries, throughout the world, we
lived communally. Having individual families siloed off from
one another behind fences, out of sight and out of mind,
is a relatively recent social structure that we accept. This
model has been forced upon us, at a steep cost to parents and
children.

What would it take to go back? Not go back in time, but
to really look back, understand other cultures—cultures
under threat of erasure, cultures subjected to force and exploitation, resilient cultures that continue to thrive despite
colonization—and glean wisdom from them. We don't need
to re-create social structures wholesale, but we could learn
more communal aspects of living, use them to rethink and
reshape American family life.

When I was younger, I was told that the United States
was a melting pot of people and cultures from around the
world. That followed the model of assimilation; vanish and

be accepted under the identity of "American," without realizing that meant "become white" and sacrifice some of who you are. Eventually we started talking about America as a "salad bowl," different elements together making a whole, without losing their distinct identities. But for many people, children of immigrants and some "white" Americans, too, it's not so simple. Our histories and ways of life have been purged from the historical record and we must deliberately seek them out.

My parents' silence spoke volumes. To this day parts of them seem like a lockbox, impenetrable to me. Do they not share because it hurts? Because it feels too complicated to explain? Or because, practically speaking, what would be the point? What good lies in revisiting difficulty and reliving it? My inheritance is a lifetime of questions, of unearthing and excavating, trying to work it all out.

IN THE FALL OF 2020, roughly seven months into pandemic life, I talked with Dani McClain, the author of *We Live for the We: The Political Power of Black Motherhood*, about how she and her family were faring. She told me that as an unpartnered parent she needed her mother, who lives nearby, to help take care of her daughter. But she added that nearly everyone she talked to, even those who were partnered or married, needed their mother—or mother-in-law, grandfather, auntie, whoever was in their support system—to survive.

"There's a way that this pandemic is revealing that two adults isn't enough . . . there's been this narrative that two adults is somehow enough for kids," McClain says. "And I think that more and more people are realizing healthy parenting means parenting in community, healthy parenting means parenting in an intergenerational environment."[5]

I suspect that most of us often find ourselves wanting more—more support, more people to share the load, more time with blood and chosen family. Covid-19 has no doubt intensified these desires, but if we're being honest, they existed long before the pandemic. When you find yourself marooned in that feeling of lack, think of William McKinley. Think of forced assimilation into a culture of individualism, no matter how "benevolent" it may seem. It isn't just colonized people who were coerced into adopting an isolated way of life; it's all Americans.

Like so many others, my family's survival relies more than ever on community—or, to put it in the dated language of the pandemic, our "pod." While we all count on distance from others to stay safe, over time we've also learned that our mental and emotional health deteriorates without others to talk, play, share a meal, and unwind with.

Even in a period of my life forever scarred by uncertainty, one thing I know unequivocally is that my family would not have survived 2020 without the Chase-Chens, another family of four: Becca and Jondou and their daughters, Ruth and Sunny, ages seven and four, the same as ours. For eight straight months, our virtual kindergarteners played together every day after school. We rotated houses and took turns picking up our toddlers, who were preschool classmates, each day.

Our relationship started simply enough—primarily as

a childcare arrangement with people we were friendly and generally vibed with. But slowly, months of daily contact—getting to know each other's children, sharing schedules and scheduling complications, learning family histories and personalities—forged a surprising, more intimate bond. They invited us to dinner at their place one Wednesday night. Then they invited us again. Within a few weeks, it became a standing date. There were so many meals together: spaghetti and meatballs, enchiladas, pizza, split pea soup, oxtails—the bones begging to be picked up and the satiny meat sucked off—in a rich broth, and stewed tomatoey white beans topped with a mountain of spiced shrimp. Over these Wednesday dinners, we weathered toddler meltdowns, election uncertainty, a few health scares, and the general stress of life.

The day rioters stormed the Capitol at the start of 2021, we talked about our fears as we set the table and pulled condiments from the fridge, our kids watching *Rescue Riders* in the other room. We hosted the Chase-Chens for Thanksgiving and Christmas Eve, when Will and I prepared a Filipino Noche Buena feast: fresh-fried lumpia, pancit bihon, pork apritada. As I looked at them across our table, it felt good knowing we were giving them the same things they'd offered us week after week. So much of pandemic life has been defined by loss and deprivation. The meals with our friends fueled a sense of abundance, a new iteration of family.

I WAS RAISED BY IMMIGRANTS WHO came to America with very little and worked their way into the middle class.

It feels shameful to admit that I don't have the desire to hustle up that same ladder, but that ambition has never existed in me, no matter how much or how long I hoped it would show up. My daughters will have fewer financial resources than I did, but I already know I have given them more of a sense of self and confidence and community than my parents, who spent years just surviving, were able to give me. "Better" or "worse" hardly feel like the appropriate ways to measure these versions of my family, but I know that I prefer the latter for my children.

"I could live only for myself, for my immediate family, following the expectations of my parents, whose survivor instincts align with this country's neoliberal ethos, which is to get ahead at the expense of anyone else while burying the shame that binds us," writes Cathy Park Hong.[6] I'll admit that pursuing the community-oriented way of life I desire still feels strange at times. What I was taught doesn't easily give way to what I want. I find myself questioning if I can trust the connections I've made with people, if they are genuine. How could people I've known only a few years possibly understand and accept the person I've always been? But when I sit, breathe, let these thoughts pass through me, I'm left with my desire to be seen by others. My need to find better ways of being in relationship persists. So that is what I go with.

Noli and Ligaya know how to spin a dreidel and swap coins accordingly; they know more about Jewish culture than I did until I was nineteen, when my freshman college roommate gave me a crash course over tins of hamantaschen sent by her mother. They have Filipinx classmates and brown-skinned teachers; for the earliest years of their lives their authority figures were mostly women who spoke English as a second language. As of now, we have absolutely no idea how we would pay for orthodontia or their college educations if they decide to go, but right now they have more than ten grown-ups in their life whom they love and trust, who see them fully, and whom I would let discipline them without a thought.

How can we show our children that even as social circles shrink, it is also possible to deepen dependence on family, neighbors, and even strangers? How can we instill the idea that all people are our people?

The American Dream is based on the idea that freedom is about being unburdened from others, having the power to do whatever we want, whenever we want. It is deeply individualistic. But, as activist Mia Birdsong explains in her book *How We Show Up: Reclaiming Family, Friendship, and Community*, there is an older understanding of freedom that we must rediscover. The words *free* and *friend* are derived from the Indo-European *friya*, which means "beloved." Freedom, Birdsong writes, was originally "the idea that together we can ensure that we have all the things we need—love, food, shelter, safety." Freedom is not an individual effort, but a collective one. "Being free," writes Birdsong, "is achieved through being connected."[7]

IN 1974 MY FATHER TOOK a job as a pathologist at a large hospital in a small town, a facility that served many throughout the area. Over the years, the hospital grew steadily—I remember the annual fundraising telethon and carnival that seemed to take over the whole town each summer, the Life Flight helicopter added when the hospital became a regional trauma center. All those years my father worked, providing for his family and banking on his children's dreams, putting his own on the back burner. It had always been his hope to move back to the Philippines and set up a clinic in his hometown.

As his community health wishes receded and the hospital continued to expand, he became disillusioned with managed health care, feeling, in his words, that he was "serving a corporation and not patients." (And this was in 1997.) During my final two years of high school, he would come home, immediately pour himself a beer from his kegerator, and pass the night in impenetrable silence, a cloud that hovered even as he was making dinner, talking, smiling. As a way of coping, my mom, whose job tending to the dying conveniently led to long hours, worked twelve- to fourteen-hour days.

When they decided to move to Washington State in 1997, my parents made a deal: my mom would take a desk job and my dad would "stop being depressed." He had never been diagnosed, but it was clear to all of us, even without any experience with therapy or mental health care, that he was stuck in a dark space. Their deal seems frankly absurd yet thoroughly plausible to me. I've learned to never underestimate the power of immigrant determination, the running stitch of necessity that has held our family together. Depression became something they could conquer, get past, move on from. It was only later that I found out my mother told him, "It's obvious I'm not making you happy, so if you want me to, I'll just leave." The cross-country move was their compromise.

My mother did take a desk job, doing intake for a hospice team rather than seeing patients in the field. My father joined a partnership of pathologists who contracted with hospitals; instead of serving one company, he'd be part of a team. He gave up the seniority he earned in Pennsylvania and signed on as an associate who would need to put in years to become a partner and owner. He started over.

What else happened when they moved to Washington State? They reconnected with Tita Vicki, one of my father's medical school classmates. It had been decades since they were colleagues, but their friendship was easily rekindled. They joined Pakikisama, the all-Filipino group at their church, and performed Simbang Gabi at the church every year at Christmas, a tradition they'd never had a chance to celebrate or share all those years in Pennsylvania. My father came home.

I WONDER: WHAT WOULD HAVE happened if the Philippines had never been colonized by Spain, and then by the United States? I probably wouldn't be here in America. I might be in the Philippines speaking Visayan or Kapampangan or Tagalog. I might be Muslim. I'd likely be living close to my extended family, grandparents, aunts and uncles, dozens of cousins whose houses I come and go from as though they were my own. Would a yaya have raised me? Would my family have maids and drivers? Would I like cooking as much as I do? Would I be a writer?

Maybe it's pointless to ask these questions. I saw a tweet from anthropologist Dada Docot that stopped me in my tracks, gave voice to a feeling that's been kicking around in my brain for a few years: "Hot take: To Filipinos saying they are their 'ancestors' wildest dreams,' what if our diasporic elders' wildest dream isn't really success and education, but homecoming?"[8]

Knowing that I cannot—and would not want to—change all the external forces that made my Filipino American family what it is, I am still struck by the idea of homecoming. What would it mean to return to my culture? A literal homecoming is impossible, but what would it mean for me, for so many of us, to find home in the parts of our culture that we have been separated from, lost touch with?

When I fantasize about this, I imagine myself complete. Instead of constantly trying to resolve disparate parts of myself, I could be whole. I might be content, my life defined more by connection and commonality than distance and difference.

In her work exploring the meaning of motherhood in Black culture, sociologist Patricia Hill Collins suggests that we might be better off abandoning the near-sacred Western idea equating the household with the family. She cites West African sociologist Christine Oppong, who believes this coupling erases women's true family roles.[9]

"Mothering was not a privatized nurturing 'occupation' reserved for biological mothers, and the economic support of children was not the exclusive responsibility of men," Hill Collins writes. "Instead, for African women, emotional care for children and providing for their physical survival were interwoven as interdependent, complementary dimensions of motherhood."[10]

Dimensions of motherhood: the words vibrate with power on the page, making me think how limited the American concept of motherhood is. Collins also cites Barbara Christian, who writes, "There is no doubt that motherhood is for most African people symbolic of creativity and continuity."[11] I love this definition, the way it counters flatness, dulled senses, and isolation with relationships, lineage, cleverness, and art.

What might we learn from the long histories of Indigenous and non-Western families? How can mothering be a way that we resist and combat the loneliness, the feeling of being burdened by our caring?

In the current whirl of life, when professional work, domestic work, and childcare are all happening simultaneously under the same roof, it is easy to feel defeated by the duties of mothering. To view a child as a nuisance—and to feel guilty for the thought. These sentiments are not indicative of personal failings. According to Andrea Landry, an Indigenous Anishinaabe activist from Pays Plat First Nation, they are the legacy of settler colonialism.

"Prior to colonization, we had children with us at all times, and that's how they learned their roles in our communities," says Landry. Children were taught by elders based on their interests. If adults noticed that a young girl was drawn to plants, the healers and medicine people would take her under their wings and mentor her. Now, occupied with work that keeps us apart from our children most days, Landry says, "we've lost sight of our children's strengths because we're so busy with capitalism and colonialism."[12]

For Landry, countering these systems means remembering they are constructions and therefore can be abandoned if they do not serve her or her child: "It's not about putting energy into colonial systems to change and dismantle them. It's about putting energy and investing time into indigenous systems and revitalizing them."

Currently my parents live in an intergenerational home with my brother, sister-in-law, three teenagers, and a labradoodle. If it was up to them, I suspect they'd like us all to live together in a compound, would be happy with a haphazard warren of rooms and hallways connecting us. I am not idealizing how they live, and I know there are difficulties, but there's a fluidness I see—the way the kids go up and down the stairs, the way my daughters, when they are there, go between the two families. My mother is active in all of our lives—she watches our littles, she drives the younger teenagers to and from soccer practice when my brother and sister-in-law have to work. Are there tensions? Yes. But there is also dependability, trust, and support that is easily asked for and offered.

Whether we are a melting pot or a salad bowl or just a dynamic, strange collection of people, one redeeming quality of America is that we might be able to pick and choose, from the rich assemblage of cultures that make up our country's population, the family values and practices that work for us. We can reject systems that are failing us and forge new ones, steeped in traditions that are still alive and well.

The psychologist Mary Pipher writes, "When generations interact, cultures tend to flourish. The different age groups inspire and energize each other. When we understand our interconnectedness, we value each other's gifts."[13]

From my mother and father, my daughters learn Tagalog and Kapampangan, they eat dinuguan, they talk and Face-Time with their great-grandmother in the Philippines. Our four-year-old's natural comedic tendencies make my father smile brighter than I've seen in years. My mother buys jigsaw puzzles to support our seven-year-old's interests, as well as to keep her brain and arthritic fingers stimulated.

When I began writing this paragraph, I first wrote that a scarcity mindset created by the American myths of exceptionalism and self-made individuals are what prevented my parents from connecting with others, from having the types of communities they deserved. But that didn't feel true. I now recognize this as a product of my own cultural conditioning. It is actually the American doctrine that stops white Americans and people with social power from being able to see themselves in anyone different or less fortunate than them. It is white America's inability—its lack—that gets in the way of progress, of dynamic community building and caring across racial and socioeconomic divisions.

In an essay about parenting teenagers during the pandemic, Carvell Wallace recounts how, after the 2016 election, his daughter and son asked him to help make sense of what had happened. His answer landed hot in my solar plexus, and I've since borrowed his words while talking to my daughters:

I told my children that one of the most important questions you have to answer for yourself is this: Do I believe
in loving everyone? Or do I only believe in loving myself
and my people? . . . I told them that their mother and
I had made our choices, but we could not decide for
them what kind of people they would be: They had to
decide for themselves.[14]

In community, life feels less exhausting, its weightiness
distributed. Not too much to bear, bolstered by love. Daily
life can be small celebrations that sustain us rather than
drudgery that depletes us.

For a long time, when I dropped off Noli at the Chase-
Chens after kindergarten, I worried that she might be a
burden. Meanwhile, when they dropped off their daughter,
grateful and almost apologetic in a nearly identical way, I
always waved them off like please, it's no big deal, get outta
here.

Building relationships can be messy and awkward. Interdependence requires real communication, empathy, sorting
through calendars and logistics. It means misunderstandings,
problem solving, asking and listening, not just popping in and
dropping off, but sometimes lingering and running late. But
I'll take pulling someone through my doorway so we can finish a conversation about our children's conflict because the
oven timer is going off and I don't want to burn the potatoes
over meaningless small talk accompanied by warm wine and
a sad fruit platter any day. I've grown to love the casual, chaotic negotiations required of interdependence. My time and

attention are not so precious that I cannot give them to another child, another adult, another family. They can be given freely because, it turns out, I have so much to give.

A FEW MONTHS AGO I brought my older daughter over to the Chase-Chens' house to sort through the "big clothes closet." Every few months, when the children are about to bust out of their clothes, they haul out a bunch of plastic bins filled with hand-me-downs from various friends and neighbors and size up. Becca had invited us to join, I suspect because she had noticed most of my girls' pants had holes on the knees and nearly threadbare seats through which you could definitely see their patterned underwear. Noli and I made a loaf of banana bread as a gesture of thanks. Jondou greeted us at their door with a baking dish—our baking dish, which last week held a lasagna we'd given them—filled with glowing green mangoes. "A friend of ours—well, it's a long story, but basically it's like a mango farm, and they send us boxes every year," he explained. We traded—mangoes for still-warm banana bread.

Noli's interest in sorting through clothes lasted just a few minutes, so she took off to play with Ruth. Becca had recently undergone knee surgery, so she lay on the bottom bunk bed and we chatted as I picked through little striped pants, kitty cat dresses, and unicorn socks. When it was time to pick up our younger girls from preschool, Jondou offered to get them both. Will had planned on picking up Ligaya, but, we thought, why not give him another half hour to himself?

Not long after Jondou left, a car pulled up outside the house. It was another friend of ours, Jen, and her son Teo. Jen had offered to bring dinner one night while Becca recovered from surgery—I was happy to see that she had brought arroz caldo, a gingery Filipino rice porridge and perfect convalescence food. We all hung out on the patio for a while, catching up as our three big kids ran around. Soon there was a lot of yelling, and there appeared Ligaya, fresh from preschool and carrying a mini cupcake, face covered in chocolate. Sunny was behind her in hot pursuit, but Ligaya refused to share. We grown-ups chatted for a little while longer, raising our own voices above the ambient noise of children screaming. When I finally loaded my children into the car—plus three shopping bags of clothes, the baking dish of mangoes, and fresh eggs from their backyard chickens—I laughed to myself at how we can't seem to show up at each other's houses without some kind of food offering. And then I thought—isn't that the way it should be?

Meal trains, playdates, and hand-me-downs are not proper substitutes for a society that provides affordable childcare, adequate wages, and time for leisure, but these patchwork solutions are precisely how so many of us survive. We will always find ways to take care of one another. When we lean into this natural, unstoppable, and very human urge, the results are expansive. And I want more.

I want more friends, more casual impromptu hangs, more dropping by with dinner, more walking and talking and advice sessions, more kids underfoot, more asking for and saying what we need, more hands to carry heavy boxes, more laughing and cackling and snorting, more children farting at the dinner table, more of what makes life messy, less painful, more sweet. I want to give and receive, to always be swapping Tupperware and food, all of us crowded together like curvy lumpen mangoes in a baking dish.

PART II

EXPLORING MOTHERING AS SOCIAL CHANGE

Smallness is subversive, because smallness can creep into smaller places and wreak transformation at the most vulnerable, cellular level.

—SARAH RUHL

5

MOTHERING INSISTS ON WORTHINESS

The house we live in used to belong to a couple named Charlton and Janice Wong, who lived here for nearly thirty years. Will and I bought the house in 2013, after spending a year living with my parents, saving money for a down payment that they also contributed to. Our home is in the exact neighborhood we wanted—diverse, with lots of Filipinx folks, close to public transportation, and our favorite discount produce stand. We don't have a yard, but there's a park one block away and we live next to an empty field. Power lines run above the field, lifted high by massive pylons—it's city property and will always stay empty. After looking at houses for months, we decided a yard didn't matter that much in the grand scheme of things. What did matter was that the house had a new roof, flooring, water heater, updated bathrooms.

We were spending nearly all of our savings and wouldn't be able to afford any renovations for a long time.

A little over a year later, on Mother's Day, I served brunch to a multigenerational Chinese American family at the restaurant where I worked as a server. When I ran the credit card at the end of the meal, the name on it read Janice Wong. Just as the family was about to leave, I asked if they were by any chance the Wongs who used to live on Beacon Hill. Within a few moments, I was hugging and thanking Charlton and Janice. As we embraced, Janice leaned in and whispered that another buyer had offered more money than us, but that she liked the letter we sent along with our offer. "I didn't think anyone would appreciate the energy of that house," she said. "But you did."

From then on, the Wongs became part of our lives. We ran into them at the park, where they still met and walked with old friends from the neighborhood. After I gave birth to our older daughter, Janice dropped by with hand-me-down clothes from her granddaughters. I loved being able to learn about their life, glean bits of information about the area.

Our neighborhood used to be fruit orchards tended by mostly Italian immigrants. The remnants of those orchards—plum, apple, and cherry trees—remain scattered throughout people's yards and public parks. During World War II, Seattle became a Boeing town and, with its location close to the factory, the neighborhood filled up with middle-class, blue-collar families, mostly white. In the 1970s and '80s, the city's growing Asian immigrant population bought homes in the area. That mix of people still existed throughout the neighborhood. Janice told us about some neighbors down the street who, for a funeral celebration, held a days-long gathering in their alley, perfuming the streets with roasted pig and other fragrant foods.

"Things are changing now, though, with white people coming and gentrification," she said. She glanced at Will. "No offense." She told us about her friend, an older Japanese woman who was confused when her new neighbors, a young white couple, knocked on her door to tell her they were having a party, to not be angry if it got a little noisy. She and her friend had laughed about it—as though they would ever call the police for a party! "Live and let live," she said. "That's the way it is around here."

The Wongs raised their children, welcomed their grandchildren, and hosted countless family meals in this house. I always assumed they updated the house to maximize its market value until Janice told me otherwise. They had actually updated it in preparation for Charlton's retirement. Since they'd be spending more time at home, and much of that time taking care of their granddaughters, they decided to make the house more comfortable. But then something unexpected happened: Charlton was diagnosed with Parkinson's disease. In the face of his inevitable and likely rapid physical decline, they had to rethink the plan they had made for the next phase of life. How long before he couldn't go up and down the stairs? Before getting in and out of the house, up and down the long driveway, would be too difficult?

After Charlton's diagnosis, their youngest son floated the idea of he and his wife selling their home and Charlton and

Janice selling theirs, and then all of them purchasing a house big enough for everyone, including their two granddaughters. And so they did, which is how we came to be the new owners of the home.

I thought of Charlton when, after my C-sections, I kept ascending and descending the stairs to a minimum for two weeks and needed to use the arm rail to steady myself. I was only temporarily disabled, but it stays with me. I think of him still when my knees, which are creaky and have a tendency to make popping sounds, make themselves heard as I head downstairs and I wonder if I am headed toward total knee replacement. When I realize that I need to turn the lights on at night when I head to bed—it's no longer enough to count seven steps to the landing and seven more to the top of the stairs in the dark. I'm getting older. We all are. The Wongs never intended to leave their home. It was the reality of aging and disability that forced their hand.

ONE BILLION PEOPLE AROUND THE world live with some form of disability. That's roughly 15 percent of the global adult population, according to the World Health Organization.[1] In the United States, about 26 percent—or one in four adults—lives with disability.[2]

"The numbers . . . suggest that disability is a common part of human life," writes artist and design researcher Sara Hendren. "An ordinary experience, infinite in variety, replete with creativity and heartbreak, from sources internal and external, and carrying social stakes everywhere."[3]

There's no single, all-encompassing definition or experience of disability. It looks and feels different for everyone. There are many types—congenital, acquired, intellectual, invisible—and ways that disability presents to others. Disability is impacted by environmental factors as well as intersecting identities. Disability—and this is the part that we so rarely consider—isn't solely defined by physical or mental impairment, but also by the way our society is organized and who is prioritized within it. As scholar and artist Sunaura Taylor states, "disability—like gender, class, and race—is a social force that affects the world in a pervasive manner."[4]

The pandemic has exposed how vulnerable we all are: just one errant droplet away from severe illness or incapacitation. No amount of exercise or dieting will prevent or ready you for contracting Covid or falling victim to a serious accident. There are no safeguards against being forced to navigate the world as a disabled person.

OUR FRIEND LEVI WAS BORN with shortened arms and fewer than five fingers on each of his hands. Once, when Levi was in Seattle for a work trip, he came over for a drink. Noli was three at the time—talkative, observant, very interested in narrating everything she was doing or thinking, sorting things into same and different. She had met Uncle Levi before, but as a much less sentient being. When they met again, I could see that she was taking stock, looking at his arms and hands. "Your hands are different," she told him.

"Yup, they are," Levi replied. She didn't say anything else.

That night I checked in with Noli about their conversation and told her that if she had any questions for Uncle Levi about his body or how he uses his hands, she could just ask him. The next day, we all set out on a long wander, eating, drinking, and exploring the alleys and streets of our neighborhood. As we walked, I mentioned the talk I had with Noli, thinking how very responsible and progressive it was of me to tell her it was okay to talk about disability and to ask someone directly about theirs. "Hope that's okay," I said, assuming it was.

"It's fine, I guess," he said. "But it's not really my job to explain myself to your kid or anyone else's."

I felt like an asshole. I thought of all the times I've been the only "other" in a room—woman, mother, brown person—and was asked to speak on behalf of so many people, be the representative. There are times when I'm willing to do it, but many others when I resent it (and often still do it, deepening my resentment). Of course it's not Levi's responsibility to educate us, no matter how much affection he might feel for my child. It's my duty to talk to her about disability, so she can show up with some basic understanding in the first place. So she knows that we care about disability because we care about people.

Why does disability seem so foreign, so difficult for able-bodied people to discuss? How did I make it nearly forty years before I started seriously considering it? That brief conversation stuck with me, prompted me to think proactively about how to talk to my kids about bodies, how we should be living in a world that makes it possible for all bodies to thrive.

Realizing I have much to learn (and unlearn) and teach my children, I wanted to understand disability, accessibility, and disability justice better.

In her book *What Can a Body Do?* Sara Hendren writes that "ability and disability may be in part about the physical state of the body, but they are also *produced* by the relative flexibility or rigidity of the built world."[5] The subtitle of Hendren's book, *How We Meet the Built World,* frames her work as interrogating how the structures we make—from sidewalks to chairs to buildings—is as much a factor in creating disability as the body a person inhabits. In other words, disability isn't always the starting point—it's the result of schools, streets, and institutions that are created without consideration of the different types of bodies that move through the world, and within a strict definition of "normal" bodies.

We believe that able-bodied people are self-sufficient and independent, but they are supported by aspects of our built environments—think stairs and flashing walk signs, which are so common we give them little thought. If architects, engineers, and designers deployed more ramps, inclines, or street signs that use audio cues, then an inability to walk up the stairs or see wouldn't be considered a significant disability. Our culture celebrates people for their independence and mobility, but the truth is that it is set up for able-bodied people and has historically banished or hidden the disabled. We worship young and docile bodies. When they are unruly or show signs of aging, they are considered problematic, and we're marketed products and services to "fix" or "solve" them.

I'm uncomfortable with the idea that able-bodied people

"give rights" to disabled folks, rather than starting from the assumption that disabled people deserve everything they need to get around as easily as possible. In the disability justice model, rights aren't bestowed upon anyone—instead disabled people are at the decision-making table, creating spaces, agendas, and institutions. Instead of talking about accommodating disability, why don't we talk about making our communities and environments accessible to everyone? How can we shift the conversation from disability to accessibility? I want a world that is as welcoming as possible to everyone, an environment that allows all bodies to move freely, at their own pace, and thrive.

Rather than see disability as a category that divides us into groups, how might I teach my children something I came late to: that it is actually a great unifier, there are more "us" than "them," abnormals than normal, distinct rather than the same, in solidarity not in competition. "Disability gathers a dimensional *we* like nothing else, because disability is no more and no less than human needfulness, both personal and political," writes Hendren.[6]

Our culture loves a binary, and we tend to view things through strict divisions—black or white, right or wrong, true or false—rather than with nuance, when two seemingly opposing concepts can be true at the same time. Able-bodied and disabled is a widely accepted binary, though it is possible to pass through one on the way to the other, to experience both throughout one's lifetime, even simultaneously. We think that able-bodied people are independent, while disabled people are wholly dependent. But this is where the binary falls short. "Our ideas about independence and dependency lead us to see the world in an either/or way," writes psychologist Mary Pipher. "In fact, we are all interdependent all of the time."[7]

DISABILITY AND AGING HAVE A similar effect on us: they create bodies with varying capabilities, new limitations and possibilities. Bodies classified this way are ones that, in mainstream American culture, are deemed less worthy and deserving. All human bodies are headed in the same direction, though, as disability justice activist Leah Lakshmi Piepzna-Samarasinha succinctly puts it: "Abled People: Time's Up. Especially Because You Will Eventually Become Us."[8]

I once saw a sign hanging outside of the senior citizen center in my friend's hometown of Pacific Grove, California. This was over eight years ago, but I still think of it often. As we went for a walk along the coast, marveling at the ocean, the fog, and the red-hot pokers, there it was, a both matter-of-fact and celebratory reminder of a universal truth: "Everybody's Doin' It . . . Aging!"

During the pandemic I let myself pass into an undeniably aging body. For almost ten years, I had dyed my hair black to cover up my gray. I stopped. Allowing my gray to flourish is an ongoing exercise in accepting myself. It's also the behavior I want to model for my daughters. I'm supposed to buy in—and have for years—to the false idea that older is less attractive, less desirable. I confront this belief daily when I look at myself in the mirror. The evidence is there: I am a woman, aging. The stark transition from black to white feels dramatic—going from visible to invisible, sometimes unrecognizable even to myself.

A classmate of my younger daughter, CJ, is always happy to see me on the preschool playground. He charges at me, grinning widely, waving and shouting, "Hi! Hi! Hi Ligaya's grandma!!" The first time it happened, I forced a laugh, but I felt sad—sad that, at such a young age, children associate gray hair with grandparents or septuagenarians but have no idea what a forty-four-year-old middle-aged woman looks like.

On good days, I consider going gray a power move that says, "Fuck you, I like me." I've noticed in my circle of friends that people often say women with gray hair are beautiful. It's not the appearance we admire, but the substance—the act of living freely. Going gray insists that the world bend to you just a little bit, that you refuse to follow the standard. My hair won't be gray, only. It will be silver, charcoal and cloudy skies, mountainsides of granite and slate, opal and onyx, plush chinchilla fur, and smoke. Not one dimension from a box—as up and down and light and dark as life itself.

Is it okay to compare disability to this aspect of aging? I'm not sure. I'm not trying to equate having gray hair with having a disability. Historically people have been institutionalized, even killed for being disabled. A little ageism hardly feels comparable. What I am saying, though, is that it is the same force—a myopic idea of which bodies are worthy—that links them, and that also creates a possibility for solidarity and deeper understanding. What would it take for us to consider both on the same plane, which is to say that neither being disabled nor growing older is a problem, just the way bodies are? Is it possible to make the mental and cultural shift to seeing difference as variations that have no inherent value?

Mothering is rooted in children's bodies. The steady rhythm of daily life, or lack thereof, shows up in their physical forms. We know that their bodies, even if they are safe for a few years, will eventually be judged as worthy or unworthy, valued or not. I watch my daughters like a hawk, memorizing the way Ligaya comforts herself by scratching her face, aggressively enough that she typically has at least one open wound at all times. I know attractive is not the most important characteristic a person can have, but I also worry about her going through life with facial scars. I am vigilant about monitoring Noli's subtle but substantial birthmark, a pool of brown skin that looks like cream poured into coffee before it is stirred, flowing over her left shoulder, into her armpit, and all the way down her arm. I watch to see if it grows or changes.

Noli is light-skinned with glowing hazel eyes, and I worry that she will pass for white, that throughout her life she will slip into whiteness to avoid conflict, to smooth out the awkward edges of certain interactions. I also worry more that she'll get comfortable there and, when convenient, assume a sense of entitlement and privilege. I worry that if she embraces and leads with her Filipinx identity, she'll be made to feel that—as mixed-race and American-born—she's not Filipinx enough. I know I am operating from a defensive standpoint, but this is the place that has helped me survive and insist on my inherent worth.

Believing in the inherent value of your body—and yourself—is a tricky act in modern America, where we are expected to work a paid job in order to "earn a living." The invention of disability has been essential in developing the modern world and our American culture of work. "Scholars have exposed the role of disability in the creation of capitalism and labor relations," writes Taylor, "particularly in contributing to definitions of a 'work-based' system versus a 'needs-based' system of distribution."[9]

Disability allows us to vilify and denigrate those of us with obvious needs while lionizing those who can and are willing to work, to give their bodies over to productivity. It allows people with power and money to say that unless you are willing and able to spend your time working outside the home for wages, you are undeserving of care and financial support. It makes the fact that health and stability are human rights somehow negotiable.

THE 2020 DOCUMENTARY *CRIP CAMP* covers, in part, the occupation of the San Francisco federal building in April 1977 by disability activists, a protest known as the 504 Sit-In. The first federal civil rights protection for people with disabilities, Section 504 of the Rehabilitation Act, was signed into law in 1973. For the law to take effect, though, regulations defining disability and discrimination had to be issued. After four years the Department of Health, Education, and Welfare (HEW) still had not done so. While activists across the country staged sit-ins to demand that HEW issue these regulations, only the San Francisco protest went on for weeks, ultimately lasting twenty-eight days. It was a critical factor in the eventual enactment of strong regulations.

The activists—including people with limited mobility, wheelchairs, and in need of assistance to do daily tasks—required robust support to live in the building with any degree of comfort. They were aided by a broad coalition of people, including the Black Panther Party. As organizer Judy Heumann recalls in her memoir, *Being Heumann: An Unrepentant Memoir of a Disability Rights Activist*, "The Black Panthers . . . pushed their way into the building with fried chicken and vegetables, walnuts, and almonds. They had brought food for all 125 of us. We gathered around, amazed, talking and laughing, clapping and cheering." The Panthers brought them food every night of the protest.[10]

In one *Crip Camp* scene, a disabled activist asks a Black Panther why they are doing what they are doing. "You are trying to make the world a better place for everybody, so we are going to feed you," the man replies.[11]

The pain and difficulties and shame that we feel about our bodies, the questions we grapple with over our worthiness, don't come from inside. A person is never inherently a problem; it is the prejudging of able-bodied, cisgender men that makes so many of us feel unworthy. It is simpler, when you feel this way, to look around and try to hoard as much power and comfort as you can get. But beyond that inclination is a chance to build solidarity: we, the othered, far outnumber the standard-bearers. Together we might build something much more powerful, based on love and inclusion, mutuality and acceptance.

"Love in action is when we strategize to create cross-disability access spaces," writes Piepzna-Samarasinha. "I've seen able-bodied organizers confused by this. Why am I fighting so hard for fragrance-free space or a ramp, if it's not something I personally need?"[12]

Piepzna-Samarasinha is writing about solidarity within the disabled community, but we can expand these ideas across many identities in order to find commonalities, just as the Black Panthers did with disabled activists. "When disabled people get free, everyone gets free. More access makes everything more accessible for everybody," she writes.[13] It's a simple idea, but also revolutionary.

This kind of logic can feel strange and unfamiliar to adults, but it comes naturally to children. Even at a young age, children have a clear sense of fairness. A group of same-aged kids might be all over the map when it comes to development, gross motor skills, and abilities. They understand this and regard it as normal. If we could preserve that perspective, we could use it as a basis for building communities that are accessible to everyone, and that operate at a pace more accommodating of the realities of having a human body. When the impulse to get free—for everyone to get free—is nurtured in them, it can grow and ignite a cultural shift. It can also help kids see the creativity inherent in the adaptations many disabled people make to move through the world.

Hendren's book is filled with examples of revisions that

disabled individuals and communities have made to their environments to improve daily life. At Gallaudet University in
Washington, D.C., the primary language of communication is
American Sign Language (ASL). Newer campus buildings are
built through an approach called DeafSpace, a set of over one
hundred design elements that emphasize the unique physical
properties of ASL, as well as assets of deafness. Tables and
benches are made of wood, rather than thick plastic, because
students often slap surfaces to get each other's attention.
Wood reverberates and carries sound waves better than plastic, which absorbs it. Glass walls create interior spaces lit by
sunshine so people can go from outside to inside easily, without their eyes adjusting to low lighting, which interrupts sign-
ing. Interior surfaces and half-walls (which establish distinct
gathering spaces without sacrificing sight lines) are painted a
shade of blue that provides clear contrast with a range of skin
tones, so hand and finger motions can be comfortably seen.[14]

My favorite adaptation chronicled in Hendren's book is
one made by Chris, a man born with a left arm and a right
limb that ends, without a hand or fingers, a few inches below
his right shoulder. Chris eschews a prosthetic arm in favor
of deploying creative combinations of his left hand, his right
limb, his feet, and his toes to perform daily tasks such as
clipping his toenails, cooking, and tying his hair into a ponytail. In order to change the diaper of his newborn son—an
activity repeated many times in one day—Chris conceived of
another low-tech solution: a rope sling that hangs from his
right shoulder to suspend his son's feet, much the same way
people hold a baby's two ankles with one hand and wipe with

the other. The design cost about ten dollars and even features soft felted wool hoops to prevent any tiny ankle discomfort.[15]

Chris's diaper-changing technique is a perfect example of disabled dancer and artist Neil Marcus's statement, "Disability is not a 'brave struggle' or 'courage in the face of adversity.' Disability is an art. It's an ingenious way to live."[16]

Mothering offers us similar opportunities each day. I'd like to show my daughters that disability is a creative way of living, that aging is not the decline of life, that both can be areas of imagination and freedom. I want them to see their bodies as never lacking or "less than," but for what they are—powerful, pulsing, ever-changing sites of play, resourcefulness, and resistance.

I don't know exactly how to do this, of course. Sometimes I feel completely out of my depth, so I counter by trying to make things as simple as possible. I try to normalize concepts that are often shrouded in silence by just talking about them. To not let things fade into the background, to name them. Pointing out the person in the book *We March* who is marching in their wheelchair, noting the bright green color of the leg braces worn by a schoolmate, and leaving some quiet space for conversation to happen, for questions to come forth. Sometimes my explanations go on too long and my kids walk away while I'm still talking. Sometimes we have a nice two-minute discussion and move on until the next time—there is always a next time. Mothering is a place to begin showing young people that all bodies are built and move differently, and how, with help and thoughtfulness, we can all live fully and exactly as we are. By never turning away from differently abled or aging bodies, we also teach children that caring for them is essential and honorable work.

Disability pushes us to look for value and worth in lives that are not particularly efficient, independent, or tidy. Rather, in Taylor's words, disability challenges us to "see the sensuality, the unruliness, the beautiful potential of alternative ways of moving through space and being in time."[17] I particularly like her emphasis on sensuality, the pleasure of leaning into the body. It can free us to just be the humans we are, instead of pursuing some idealized version of humans we might never actually be.

As I age, the more convinced I am that the concept of "normal" is the most toxic thing in our culture. Anyone who isn't a straight cis white able-bodied guy learns early on that they are somehow abnormal. Our concept of what a person is— our laws, our standards for science and medicine, our very concept of "health"—is based on those bodies. Accepting and owning what distinguishes us from the "normal" who only comprise a small portion of humans on earth is liberating. We can begin speaking into existence the world we want to see: instead of telling our children to prize whiteness, purity, rationality, youth, and achievement, we can emphasize color, the need for darkness, the richness of nuance, imperfection, emotions, stillness, and age.

ON JEJU ISLAND IN SOUTH Korea, it's the skills of a particular set of older women who enrich the culture: the free divers who collect oceanic delicacies that are sold at markets and to restaurants. These women are called haenyeo, and the majority of them are over sixty. In recent years, even as the number of working haenyeos has dwindled, they have become a tourist attraction. People come from Korea and all over the world to see them work, spending long periods diving deep into frigid saltwater, then resurfacing with urchins and abalone. In 2016, UNESCO designated the haenyeo an intangible Cultural Heritage of Humanity.

A few years ago I ripped an article out of *Hemispheres,* the United Airlines in-flight magazine. I saved it in a file folder of random inspiration that I keep. A few months into growing out my gray, I found myself thinking about the haenyeo, so I dug the article out. The corners of the pages were starting to yellow.

"*Haenyeo* peak in their fifties, when they've accumulated enough experience to sense minute changes in the current," the article states. In the words of one woman: "You learn to be calm." I read the lines that caused me to tear the article out: "Visitors to Jeju see women well into their 80s and 90s abandon their walkers at the shore and seemingly morph into mermaids. . . . Youth appears to offer little advantage."

During the first fall of the pandemic, Noli's best friend lent us a children's book, *The Ocean Calls: A Haenyeo Mermaid Story,* all about the women divers of Jeju Island.[18] Little Daeyon is scared of going below the surface of the water, but is encouraged to overcome her fears by her grandmother, a haenyeo who cooks her abalone porridge. Daeyon is nurtured and protected by a group of old women who are masterful at doing something she can barely summon the courage to try. I tear up every time I read the story, moved that in the world of this book being a senior citizen is aspirational.

Do I fear my own aging body? Well, yes—but what about it do I look forward to? An increasing intimacy and familiarity and, I hope, tenderness with it. As I get older, I desire to trust my body, let it take over, to take my cues from it. How bad could nature and inevitability really be?

I actually hated dyeing my hair, staining my skin—the backs of my ears, the webbing between my thumb and index finger, the spot where the gloves that come with the box are weak—and the stray splatters on my bathroom wall, constant reminders of my delusional vanity. I always low-key resented "having" to do it, but I come from a long line of hair dyers—both my grandmothers, my mother, four out of my mom's five sisters, all of my aunts on my dad's side—seemingly all of whom have offered their (negative) opinions on my gray. I know how rare it is to see a Filipina woman who doesn't dye her hair. It stings a little when a family member tells me I look old, but I know that I like myself more than I care about what they think. I tell myself I am pressing on past the colonial standards of beauty that confine the women of my family, that threaten to confine me.

"Maybe you should dye your hair," my mother said to me once while I was growing out my roots. "After all, you should look younger than me."

At seventy-five, my mom looks amazing. She's spry and energetic. I hold my tongue and don't say what I am thinking: No matter how young she looks, no one is going to mistake me for her elder.

ULTIMATELY THE WONGS FOUND A large, modern home in a nearby neighborhood that met their needs: Charlton and Janice lived on the lower floor, their son and his family above. They were comfortable and cared for as Charlton's life became more difficult to manage and he moved to an elder care facility. He passed away two years ago, just before the Covid-19 pandemic. "In some ways, I'm relieved," Janice tells me. "What could life have been like for him if he was all alone, and we couldn't have visited him? What sort of a life is that?"

I still see Janice around, almost daily this past spring when I started walking my daughter to her final two months of kindergarten, which were happening in-person after seven months of being online. Most days our walk coincided with Janice's morning walk with Yumiko, a ninety-seven-year-old woman whose perfectly manicured rosebushes are a block from our house. Seeing her with Yumiko, a little hunched over and shuffling and moving at the same slow pace that Charlton once did, made me realize how closely Janice has lived to disability, how easily she adjusts her pace to walk arm-in-arm with those she loves, who have been decelerating for years.

"Of course, ultimately ageism is a prejudice against one's own future self," writes Mary Pipher.[19]

Now when I walk with an elder or I walk with my child, I am less irritable about having to come down to their rhythm. I think of Janice, how these little tedious journeys are an opportunity to slow down, to notice the new chartreuse tips on the spruce trees, to get lost in the brief reverie of a moment, to come to someone else's eye level and perspective, to see the world differently, if only for a few minutes. I think about how it is possible—necessary—to take care of the people our children are becoming, their future selves, right now.

6

MOTHERING AS ENCOURAGING APPETITES

As a kid, I padded into our yellow linoleum kitchen at all hours to take scoops of rice from the rice cooker that lived on the counter. I'd fill a bowl then pour patis and lemon juice over it, or soy sauce and lemon juice, depending on my mood, and eat it while sitting on the floor. My brothers used to yell at me for what they considered my highest crime, worse than being a tattletale: I'd beat them to a loaf of supermarket bakery French bread and dig out the squishy insides, which I'd chase with a shot of pickle juice straight from the jar. When they opened the paper bag, they'd find only a long, hollowed-out crust. I'd help myself to slices of Pepperidge Farm German Chocolate Cake, which my mom kept in its box in the freezer. I liked how, after eating approximately half the slices, the box had enough room to store the knife inside of it, where it would get finger-numbingly cold. My appetite has always felt outsized, and I've only ever wanted to indulge it.

Growing up, I noticed the food we ate was the product of a lot of work. Not only did it require ingredients that most people around me had never heard of, but those ingredients took a long time to cook. I was a small-town '80s kid, growing up at a time when the "ethnic" aisle in the grocery store was stocked with little more than La Choy soy sauce and canned water chestnuts. I could never imagine I'd live where I do now, shopping at Fou Lee, Seafood City, Viet-Wah, Uwajimaya, 99 Ranch, and H Mart. Many pantry staples—fish sauce, fifty-pound bags of rice, bagoong, sotanghon noodles, cane vinegar—were procured in Chinatown when we visited my Tita Fe in New York City. I remember my dad loading the hefty woven sacks of rice into the back of our van. When we arrived home, he would cut open a sack with a steak knife, flip it over, and pour its contents into our green rice dispenser, a three-foot-tall item I was oddly proud of our owning. It dispensed rice in three-cup increments with just the push of a finger.

We also ate a fair amount of canned corned beef in those days, but all the important food—the food my parents liked the most, the food we ate on special occasions, or the nights when my mom was home from work early—was Filipino. Pinakbet, munggo, adobo—dishes that required time to poach and shred chicken, braise pork belly, or chop small mountains of vegetables. For bulalo and sinigang and kare kare, we needed hours to braise pork neck bones and oxtails. When she made lumpia and pancit, typically for parties and gatherings, my mother would pull out gallon containers of Wesson oil and two electric woks and turn what seemed like laundry baskets of noodles using all her arm strength. Instead of our usual white six-cup rice cooker, she'd get out the fancy cream-colored ten-cupper with the built-in lid and decorative pastel flowers. On these occasions, I often ate so much that I got a stomachache. At age forty-four, it's not so different. I always want more: another bite, another serving, another round.

My husband likes to tell the story of the first time he came to dinner at my parents' house. There were four of us, and my mom and dad served a dinner of salad, pancit, baked salmon, and white rice. Plus two racks of smoked pork ribs. Filipinx elders are always asking you if you've eaten, always telling you to eat more. They are also the first people to declare, immediately upon seeing you, "You got fat!" The question I've been asked most frequently throughout my life by family is probably, "Have you eaten yet?" Whatever my answer is, the reply is "Kain na!"

At my home now, our oldest daughter loves chili, specifically the bean-and-beef-filled one her father makes in our slow cooker, suffusing the house with the scent of cumin. She has been known to house three consecutive bowls—topped with shredded cheddar, diced onions, crushed tortilla chips, and sour cream—in one sitting. On more than one occasion she has excused herself after one bowl to run to the bathroom and poop, ensuring she has room for another serving. I resist the urge to tease her about it because, honestly, I get it.

Our most popular family dinner is one that Will and I used to cook for ourselves when we wanted a weeknight to feel like a special occasion. We'd get a whole mackerel—usually just $2.99 a pound, so cheap for such an oily and luxurious fish—and throw it on the grill, stuffed with lemon slices and green onions. We'd have big servings, then pick at it leisurely, leaving enough leftovers to make mackerel cakes the next day. Soon after we started cooking it for our girls, we had to start buying two fish for each meal.

FOR A LONG TIME, I thought of my body as very inconvenient. Not necessarily fat, but definitely a little too much. A little too brown, a little too round, my calf muscles large, skinny jeans tight around them, decidedly indelicate. My mother commented that I was big-boned—compared to her delicate wrists, which I could loop my fingers around, my joints were thicker.

Where did I come from?

I don't know when exactly I realized that my boobs were big, but by the time I was in high school I was wearing a DD, and the soft proto-bras that had gotten me through up to that point were not going to be enough. My mother, who bought A- and B-cup bras almost exclusively from clearance racks, didn't know that you could be properly measured to fit a bra. My breasts seemed to confuse her. "You must have gotten those from your Ima," she'd say, referring to my paternal grandmother.

Other parts of me also seemed to confound her. When my leg hair started showing up, my mother said she never had enough body hair to warrant shaving. "Asian people don't have to shave," she said. After I got my period and seemed to bleed through all my panties, I wanted to try tampons, the ads for which I'd seen on TV and in magazines. "I don't know about those, we just use pads," offered my mother. My body was not a petite, hairless, familiar, Filipina body that my mother understood. I had to figure it out on my own. I drove myself to Walmart and set out in the aisles to find proper breast support in the form of the Playtex 18 Hour Bra—heavily starched, white, appropriately clinical, and able to tame my boobs into objects high and pointy.

I came from my mother's body, I got this body from her. But what do you do when your body looks nothing like hers? When she doesn't know how to help you? I don't blame my mother for not knowing to take me to the lingerie department and get measured—it would have meant focusing on parts of our bodies that she was told not to speak about, to hide. I don't consider my childhood experiences traumatic, but the lack of support and guidance certainly made body acceptance a long, emotionally turbulent process. I think of people who are deprived of meaningful bodily care early in life and the psychological damage forced upon them.

It pains me to imagine children without someone to help guide their understanding of their bodies—how good they are at keeping them alive, no matter what they look like. It hurts me to think that my mother never had that, never thought that I might need it. I was left feeling alone, a bad fit for the place I lived. I spent my adolescence wandering around feeling like loose ground meat and bits, sausage in search of a casing.

What spares someone like me from developing an eating disorder or a lifelong habit of dieting? I have no idea, but I am grateful to Baby Angela because she at least knew that she was never interested in limiting herself. I decided that being a little fat was the price I paid for always wanting seconds. I don't know why I didn't shrink myself, only allowed myself to expand, both in size and in personality.

SINCE THE MOMENT LIGAYA WAS born, people have been telling me that she looks just like me. "Your twin!" more than a few people have remarked. To me, she looks like herself, but four years in I can finally concede that there is a strong resemblance between us. Why was I hesitant to admit it?

As Ligaya grows into her own person, I see that her face looks very much like mine, but also that her body shape seems to echo mine. I don't think she'll be tall, but she will be robust and sturdy, her legs short and strong. I've never wanted to give voice to the resemblance for fear that it will curse her to have the same baggage and body image issues I've struggled with: self-conscious about her round stomach, thick calves, big boobs.

I feel less certain parenting her. With Noli, whose temperament is quite even-keeled, I feel confident and fairly objective. But Ligaya, who runs hot, is too much my familiar. That seems unfair, because she is not me, and yet I can't distance myself. When I see her dig in, stubborn, then want to turn it around but not be able to because of pride, just dig in further and scream, I'm not sure what to do. Whether to try to comfort or let her get it all out. If I knew how to manage the urge to be your worst self around those closest to you to prove you are unlovable while desperately wanting to be loved and accepted, I might have solved all my life problems years ago.

I have curiosity too: Will she, like me, have uneven body hair, her right armpit hairy and her left scattered with just a few thin wisps? Will her leg hair grow only to the middle of her shins, as though she's wearing hairy mid-calf-length socks? Will her lips stay plump and delicious and will she retain the same expressive face that makes it nearly impossible to hide her emotions?

Everyone has their own innate understanding of how to be in their bodies, including my daughters. I am trying my best to stay back, to find the delicate place where my fears exist and where they become projections I put on my children. I keep my eye out for that line so I don't cross it. I'm figuring out how to release control, follow their lead. I want to get out of their singular life paths, but I want to get in the way of the dominant narrative, box it out. How do you care and lead and recede at the same time?

Can I inspire my girls to not care what their stomachs are shaped like? To know that they are much more than their bodies? To pursue their appetites and, in the words of Carmen Maria Machado, "manifest the audacity of space-taking"? Can I give them what Machado calls "fatness of the mind"?

Caregivers play an essential role in the development of young brains and bodies that do not hold disdain for themselves. If our mothering does not equip a child to accept and respect their body, it may lay the groundwork for negative feelings that will impact not only that child, but others upon whom they will project their beliefs.

I want my daughters to unapologetically glut themselves and take up space, follow their hunger, curiosities, and desires—and encourage those they love to as well. "The unapologetic fat body is dangerous because it suggests that there's another way—and that there has always been another way," writes Machado. "So the fat mind, too, is dangerous. It, too, suggests another path."[1]

OUR BABYSITTER PENELOPE SHOWS UP one day in a T-shirt that reads, "You were brainwashed into thinking European features are the epitome of beauty." I resist the urge to hug her. I cannot resist, at the end of the afternoon, asking Noli, a beginning reader, if she has read Penelope's T-shirt. She has, but only as far as "thinking."

"I wanted to get into it with her," Penelope tells me, "but I wasn't exactly sure how."

"Should we get into it now then?" I ask.

Noli reads the shirt aloud, and we offer help as she sounds out and stumbles over letters and words. We do our best to explain what "brainwashing" is. I get her placemat off the dining room table—a laminated map of the world—and she identifies Europe, the Philippines, and Nigeria, where Penelope's family is from. We explain that, generally, people from these countries have darker skin—brown and black. In Europe, they are mostly white. We say white people who have been in power have created a culture that says that being beautiful means being thin and white. "And pointy!" Noli chimes in. I tell her that beautiful is not the most important way to be, but also that there are so many ways to be beautiful—having brown skin, a bridgeless round nose, or freckles and curly hair like Penelope.

I don't know how much she will take away, and I see that we've maybe pushed things a little longer than she would prefer. But I'm glad to be talking about it, and to be talking about it with someone my daughter loves and admires and whose relationship to her has very little to do with me.

ONLY NOW CAN I SEE that in youth I was worried about being fat because that was the only language I had for the discomfort I felt in my body. My vocabulary and understanding were so limited. I didn't have the words to say that my body felt foreign, hopelessly different, inscrutable, solitary.

It was an overall otherness that bothered me. Size was just the easiest thing to pin it on, the one reinforced by culture, within my own family. A feeling that the form I was in just wasn't quite right, always at odds with the other bodies in the room. Where I grew up, white bodies. When I went back to the Philippines, where I was *really* from, it was too big, too American, too keen on getting dark, too bossy. Nowhere was I seen as small and sweet, which even though I knew I was not and didn't want to be, still left me tender.

Opting out of traditional beauty and body standards was not a function of any felt superiority or confidence or moral high ground. It had more to do with being fully aware of how outside of it all I was. There was no way I was ever going to fit in, so I gave up. It was too much work. Even if I conformed, I wouldn't fit in, so why bother? Why stifle my appetites when winning acceptance was impossible anyway?

Since I couldn't be beautiful, I would be interesting. More than a body. Smart. Outspoken. Determined. There was a world out there, and I wanted to experience it, gobble it up, make it mine. Expand my consciousness—grow to meet it. I didn't have the words for what I was doing at the time, but nearly thirty years later while reading Virginia Sole-Smith's *The Eating Instinct*, I find language that helps me understand.

"I do believe that it's possible for anyone—infant, child, teenager, adult—to sense their own hunger and fullness, and to eat on their own terms, for both pleasure and health," Sole-Smith writes. "And, in doing so, move toward valuing their bodies for reasons beyond the aesthetic."[2]

Eating is a necessity. Being beautiful is not. Being attractive always felt unfeasible and the pursuit of it depressing, but giving in to my particular appetites, especially a love of Filipino food, gave me a sense of pride, enjoyment, and identity. It helped me to take up space.

Since childhood, my favorite special occasion dish has been pancit palabok, made of rice noodles drowning in a briny orange gravy and topped with pork, hard-boiled eggs, scallion, and, for extra salt and crunch, chicharron. My parents sometimes add a tin of smoked oysters. The sunset-colored sauce is traditionally made from pounded shrimp heads and annatto seeds, neither of which were easy to obtain forty years ago in rural Pennsylvania. In a stroke of immigrant ingenuity, they made do with what they had: cans of Campbell's Cream of Shrimp soup concentrate.

Cream of Shrimp was my private lesson in adaptability—making do with what you have, being okay with what is in hand. It also showed me persistence and pride. Our family's life was so different from my parents' childhoods, but even as they assimilated, they never let go of home, not really. They made their life here, including the food, their own. My parents' dishes were approximations, built on shadow flavors and memory. But that didn't stop us from lapping it all up. Over the years, grocery store selection got better—my mom started using chayote squash instead of zucchini in her tinola. She added leaves plucked from pepper plants during the summer and stashed in the freezer for future use.

When I visited the Philippines, I learned what these dishes were "really" supposed to taste like: tongue-stripping sour of green mangoes, saline and shuddering funk of bagoong. Bananas I'd never seen before—some not much bigger than my fingers—soft and buttery and always on the verge of collapsing, sweeter and fuller in my mouth than any banana I'd ever tasted. Mangoes yellow and bursting, sun-warmed stringy fruit disintegrating in my mouth, juice dribbling down my chin, sucking the yellow and black bruised skin clean. Leaving a hollowed cup of flesh on the table. Each bite was like coming into my birthright—everything I wanted and craved and deserved but didn't even know I could ask for.

At home—in the kitchen, at the dining room table, in Pennsylvania, in the Philippines—I was learning who I was—literally ingesting it, making it a part of me. This pursuit has outlasted every other ideal I was force-fed or shown. It tastes and feels more satisfying than being considered pretty. I, and so many other girls and women, were told that if we tamed our appetites, we'd be more appealing. But to whom, and for how long?

My tongue, my body—they're pleasure-seeking missiles launched the day I was born, and that I have no idea how, and no desire, to shut down. On each visit to the Philippines, the food would come, made by others, served steaming hot and placed on the lazy Susan in the middle of Ima's table. One dish, one side was never enough—three or four dishes at a time, always a fried fish, always rice, always fresh fruits. To me it felt like a lavish buffet—and it was, humble ingredients transformed, through skill and time, into luxurious food: burong isda, a paste of fermented fish and rice, sour and stinky and pungent; dinuguan, organ meats braised in pigs' blood, made tart and fiery with vinegar and chiles; bulalo, the richest broth made with slow-cooked oxtails, overflowing with large bones, unripe bananas, and potatoes.

I'll never forget when, at a family party, I made myself a little dish of saw saw, a kind of personalized dipping sauce, to accompany a bowl of bulalo. The saw saw was made of patis and fresh kalamansi juice. I used it to flavor each spoonful of soup, to cut through the fattiness of oxtail; I savored it, let it roll over my tongue. I felt eyes on me and saw my Tito Albert watching me with a smile. He turned to my dad, smacked him on the arm, pointed at me, and said, "Talagang Pilipina." Truly Filipina.

At the time it was validation I desperately wanted. I had not yet realized that I always was and always am truly Filipina. That there is no test one has to pass, no measure of authenticity or purity. I am Filipina enough because I am Filipina. And what made me feel seen and recognized as the Pinay person I wanted to be seen as was the very activity that had always felt so fraught for me: eating. Of course, it wasn't just me that made it fraught. A culture that prizes thinness and whiteness did that. Add to that the American colonial legacy in the Philippines: a country of brown people convinced they could only be attractive if they made themselves white. It's not just sinister, it's impossible.

"They say that beauty is in the eye of the beholder and that ugly is as ugly does. But these are lies. Ugly is everything done to you in the name of beauty," writes Tressie McMillan Cottom. "Knowing the difference is part of getting free."[3]

I am my parents' child for sure, but a distorted, bloated, American version of the one they expected. My body, my appetites, my ambition distended beyond their imagination and, I sometimes fear, their comprehension. I spent so many years trying to make sense of my body, alone, but somehow I always had my fat mind.

MOTHERING OFFERS US AN OPPORTUNITY to form new relationships with our bodies, to listen to them. It is through tuning in to our physicality that we caregivers can fully access our power. We have so many opportunities to show children that they are not alone in navigating the murky waters of what a body should be like, how we might treasure it, and how we should care for and nourish it.

My mother used to stand in front of her full-length mirror in her underwear and shake her belly. The skin was pale, textured like crepe paper, beautifully soft to the touch, but she shook it with disgust, chanting "flabby flabby flab." She gardened in long-sleeved shirts and a visor, and she chided me for sitting in the sun. I didn't listen, so there was always a tension: I was inherently a little disobedient. I went with it. But it's not so simple: I wasn't bad and she wasn't wrong, we were both just following the stories we knew. I happened to be born into a culture where there were a few more scripts available. I saw other ways of being that seemed better suited to me. I want to give my daughters even more options.

Right now the little one loves her body. She likes to be naked, to show off her booty butt. She is loved on for her roundness, a personality defined by fullness, a robust sense of self and humor and confidence. She has never had a problem expressing herself. On the day she was born I offered her a pacifier, which she immediately spat out and, as if for comic effect, continued dramatically spitting and coughing. She is naturally funny and physical, rough-and-ready, clear about her desires and what she will not abide.

Now, we sit down to the two mackerels that will feed our family of four. It's a bony fish, so we still sift through the meat for Ligaya, separating meat from the tinik. She eats breathlessly, cleaning the plate as quickly as Will can get more fish on it. We used to give her one eyeball from each fish, Will or I eating the other, but now she insists on eating all of them, denying us the delicacies we used to relish. She loves the eyeballs, just like her Apu, my dad, who breaks bones at the table with his teeth to suck the marrow, who won't let a single organ or bit of gristle go to waste. Noli, just like my mother, wants the crispy skin, the part that is most charred, flaky, and salty. I see my parents in my children's eating habits, and I'm glad they are here to see it too.

My mother makes them adobo, I make them pancit on their birthdays. They like sinigang but just the meat and sour broth and rice—no okra or eggplant yet. This is the food we are passing down to them. Also: kalbi, pad Thai, oysters and clams plucked straight from the cold waters of the Puget Sound, kielbasa and sauerkraut, kimbap, dim sum turnip cakes and taro-wrapped sticky rice, frozen mandarin orange chicken from Costco, Maruchan instant ramen, homemade burgers, refrigerator soup made from CSA vegetables wilting in the crisper. I try to never deny them seconds or thirds, to let them figure out when they are full, to trust their bodies, something I am still working on.

On our tenth wedding anniversary, I dig a few old photos of Will and me out of plastic boxes to share with our girls. I like to remind them that we were people before we were Mama and Daddy. There's one that makes me laugh out loud—from our first big vacation together, two years after we met: ten days in Mexico, traveling by bus from Mexico City along La Costa Esmeralda, then to Oaxaca to meet friends. It's printed on cheap photo paper, corners of the image peeling off, a date of 9/10/2009 in the right-hand corner. We were on the beach in Veracruz, and a photographer was wandering around offering to take and print photos. I wanted a souvenir. We were facing west during that golden glowing hour just before sunset—the kind of light that makes everyone look gorgeous—the waves behind us, ankle deep in warm salt water.

The photo is ludicrously overexposed. My face looks bronze—literally like polished metal—and Will's white chest is nearly translucent, any definition or trace of his nipples and abs totally washed out. We howled with laughter when we got it; it looks like I am vacationing with a ghost. I show it to my daughters, assuming they will see what I see and we can all laugh at Daddy.

Instead Noli takes one look at it and says, "Mama, did you get fat?"

I want to hide, to disintegrate into the mattress we are all lying on. I only have a second to decide what to do.

"Yes."

"Yeah, Mama, your belly got real fat," agrees Ligaya.

"Yup," I say, feigning nonchalance. "Bodies change, sometimes they get bigger or fatter, sometimes they get smaller. It doesn't really matter what our bodies look like, though—what matters is that they keep us alive. I think mine is doing a good job." I know this is true, just as I know I am saying this to myself as much as them. Can they tell?

"Mama's exactly right," Will chimes in. I am grateful for this, even as I resent his body, which is as lean and wiry as it was the day we met.

"Yeah, you definitely got fatter," says Noli. "But I like your fat belly because it's squishy and kind of like a pillow."

I want to be humiliated by this, if only because it would

feel familiar. Trying out new feelings with these small people I made, who I am responsible for guiding, feels like growth, which is so uncomfortable, even though I've imagined a moment like this and hoped I could rise to the occasion.

"Well, my belly has only gotten bigger since I grew you two in there," I say. The truth is that my whole body seems to have gotten bigger over the last decade, as has my appetite.

I still don't have full sensation in my lower abdomen, the result of two C-sections. When I gave birth to Ligaya, I spent nearly an hour shaking and shivering uncontrollably (normal, I was told) as a very meticulous obstetrician removed all of the scar tissue from my first surgery (apparently there was a lot) before sewing me together. The fundamental shape of my midsection has morphed from tapered at the waist to something rectangular and vaguely refrigerator-shaped. It seems that this weighty area of my body will always be slightly numb, and I deal with this mostly by trying to be numb about it too. But my children force me to see it, and to see it differently.

I look down at my stomach. It is fat. I've done a good job, though, I think. To my girls, fat is just fat, an adjective. It's only me who brings judgment to it. Suddenly, before I can ruin the moment by speaking, they are on me, kissing my stomach, resting their faces on it, petting it, squealing.

"My only Mama, my squishy Mama," Noli sings. Ligaya blows raspberries that make me laugh and gasp for air. They catch me off guard, get me out of my head. In this moment I am delighted to be in my body—this soft, scarred, miraculous, confounding, life-giving body.

7

MOTHERING TOWARD MOVEMENT

Chris, a nine-year-old girl, rocks bath and forth, her head tilted toward the fluorescent lights above. As she sways to and fro, she bangs on a rattle. My four-year-old, listening to Drake in the living room, moves her juicy hips from side to side, singing "passionate from miles away" over and over. My thirteen-year-old niece, high energy and an avid soccer player, likes to end each day curled up in bed, rubbing the silken corner of an old blanket in her palm. Young people know their internal rhythms, how they like to move their bodies.

I've never met Chris—an intellectually disabled girl, also partially deaf and blind. Aspects of her life were recorded by sociologist David Goode, who spent decades observing nonverbal children. After several months with Chris, Goode manipulated his own body—covering his left eye, plugging his ears, and simulating Chris's actions—in order to try to discern why she moved as she did. He concluded that Chris's physical efforts provided her "otherwise impoverished perceptual field with a richness her eyes and ears could not give her." She found gratification in using the parts of her body available to her. Goode writes that he was, and still is, "struck by the inventiveness in this activity."[1]

While rocking and rattling may not seem like worthwhile activities to some people, disability scholar Sunaura Taylor insists that Chris makes us consider the experiences that each of us, in our different bodies, are capable of. Chris's movements are "deeply pleasurable and meaningful, even as they remain hidden or even unknowable to the rest of us."[2]

When I read this, my response is physical. My hands feel warm and tingly. Yes. All beings are capable of sensual experiences that are significant to them. Going for a long run in the sun; hitting the gym for a powerlifting session; paddling smoothly in a kayak, barely disturbing the surface of water; doing booty drops in the club when the DJ plays your jam; rocking back and forth with a rattle: these activities might be nothing alike, but they all hold value and meaning to the people doing them. In a world that tells us to move in pursuit of a better body, for maximum health, I am convinced that it is precisely these hidden, unknowable pleasures that should be our motivation to move.

MY HUSBAND HAS WHAT I call "squirrel energy." If he doesn't break a sweat each day, he is noticeably irritable or gives off weird vibes that make it hard for me to be around him. I am a sloth in comparison. I could happily spend hours each day lying down. But that doesn't mean I don't crave activity. In fact, I love to move my body, to fully inhabit it as it bends, folds, stretches, and turns.

Movement is vital, as is rest. How each of our bodies prefers to move is an expression that is individual and complex, influenced by where we are raised and by whom, as well as what activities we are exposed to. At some point in childhood many people, myself included, receive the message that their bodies are suitable or unsuitable for different pursuits. That we're not strong or disciplined enough. We internalize those ideas, and they affect how we approach our physicality. We doubt our capabilities, have less tolerance for the awkward fumbling required in learning. We might only pursue activities that we know we'll be good at relative to our peers. We accept someone else's vision of our bodies and close ourselves off to so many experiences.

When I was a kid, my parents signed me up for soccer. My team was called the Ponies. I went to practices, but when I was subbed in during our first game, I started crying and didn't stop until they let me leave the field. I tried gymnastics, basketball, and softball—I stuck with these longer, but mostly begrudgingly. I scored a total of one point during my eighth-grade season of basketball; I made two free throws but stepped over the line on the second one. I loved dancing and took ballet classes for years, but around age twelve my teacher told me that I was not the type of girl who would ever be a real ballerina and focused her attention on the tallest, most slender girls.

Once I was old enough for movement to cease to be a mandatory extracurricular, I stopped with regular sports. Exercise wasn't something people in my house did—I've never seen my mother or father run, and they certainly didn't play tennis or racquetball. From what I could tell, they cleaned the house and drank beer, respectively, in their downtime. I settled into other activities: reading, playing the piano, performing, writing.

I didn't dance in any formal setting or studio for years. Take me to a house party, though? I'd tear it up, sweating like I'd just played four quarters of NBA basketball. I knew my movements were a lot for some people, but I had my friends shaking it right there with me. Also, I was too high on endorphins—or, for a few years, too drunk—to care. One of my favorite places on earth is the dance floor at a wedding reception—let me take Uncle Clarence for a spin, do the electric slide, be one of the last few people barefoot on the dance floor when "Like a Prayer" comes on and we're all clapping our hands above our heads. Dancing was a special occasion, night-out kind of thing, set apart from everyday life. It took me nearly twenty years to find my way back to it, which is a shame because it is one of the loves of my life.

In *The Eating Instinct*, Sole-Smith considers how we might rediscover our particular appetites. She is writing about food, but when I take in her words, I immediately think of dancing:

"Recognizing ourselves as capable eaters means identifying the factors that caused us to lose that identity in the first place—the particular mix of biology, psychology, socioeconomic positioning, and life experience that is different for everyone. It means reclaiming control of our bodies." That reclamation isn't one-step: it's a process of self-discovery, one that might evolve over months, years, a lifetime.

"The only way to learn to eat is by eating," concludes Sole-Smith. The same is true of movement.

When I hit thirty, I was frankly offended that my body, which had been fine on a movement regime of walking the city, seemed to require more to stop itself from expanding. I spent a few years half-heartedly trying to find an exercise routine that worked for me: something low-effort that would give me the exact results I wanted, without my having to change any other aspect of my life. Running didn't work—I could stop whenever I wanted, and I never stopped thinking about the minutiae of daily life while I was doing it. I liked the rigor and heat of Bikram yoga, the way I'd settle deeper into poses and, over time, find peace in the place my body couldn't progress past. But it was expensive and the prescribed sequence of poses, which never changed, felt rigid.

I started going to a movement class called Dance Church a few months after giving birth to my older daughter, and I kept going through the entirety of my second pregnancy three years later. I have been going for more than six years; it's the longest I have ever stuck with any form of exercise or movement. Before the pandemic I went every week, sometimes two or three times a week. The class consists of guided improvisation set to pop music, taught by professional dancers, but open to people of all bodies and abilities. There are no mirrors, so you can't look at yourself. When you see your movements reflected back at you, it's in someone else's body. Directions are called out, part aerobics, part Lisa Frank poetry: *rainbow arms, reach and pull, sparkle rain, put it in your pelvis.*

Dance delivered me, week after week, back to myself, restoring a sense of command and humor in my body that I mostly only ever felt slipping away. Synovial fluid sliding around, a little burr of heat and pleasure in the arch of my foot, a tiny but not painful pop in my right knee, an openness in my right hip that I don't want to push lest it rip me open and a river of lava pour out. I'd never been in touch with my body like this, never writhed so safely and uninhibited. I did it just for myself, but it gave me unexpected relationships, pleasure I didn't know I needed.

What I love most are the people in class who are just fucking going for it—not only in big bombastic moves, but small quiet ones too. My favorite thing in the world is seeing someone move and knowing that only they could have done that particular movement in that particular moment. Our brains and bodies are engaged, but it's not in self-conscious or even rational thought. It's flow, it's vibes. This is what our bodies are for, I remember thinking one night in class. They are here to say something, without words. I want to lean in closer to people, to listen. To look more closely, so as to hear.

Maybe it's because I've staked my living on words that the communication dance offers feels so significant. I love a well-crafted sentence, a description that somehow lands in the body and is impressed on the mind forever. But just as much I love the way Cayla, a person I always find myself dancing next to, squats down and, her dreamy ass leading the way, turns her body like some deep oceanic current. Her arms, raised above her shoulders, and her delicate neck, curved like a summer squash flourishing in the heat, tell me that she is free.

The choreographer Bill T. Jones remarked that in our culture of incessant talking, "we're constantly trying to convince the world that there's beauty in movement. That space is an eloquent medium. That text is not always necessary."[3]

At the start of every Dance Church, I anticipate the arrival of a wave. I'm feeling my way into my body, its tight and tender parts, and feeling the heat in the room build. That vitality, shared and created by dozens of people, collects and crescendos into a force that lifts and propels me. Inevitably, at some point I exit my brain completely and am just a body, a body with so many others. I am movement, salt water, energy: I have become the wave.

Zadie Smith once said that, for her, dancing was an antidote to what increasingly feels like a condition of modern life: having an online profile, a persona, personal brand. For those of us who grow resistant to or tired of performing ourselves, movement offers an escape. "I feel most free dancing among strangers," Smith said. "To me, individuation is a kind of hell; the most human thing is to be part of people, less aware of the self."[4]

For over a year, I danced with a woman whose arms and hips created a circle of light around her. She wore her long black braids around her head like a crown, painted her lips in dark brownish-purple lipstick, and wore big dangly earrings. She knew how to show up. I wanted to know her, but it was enough just to receive her energy, lock eyes, and groove together from across the room. I have no idea exactly when or why we started talking, but within a minute, I learned that this woman, Dalya, was Filipinx and Egyptian, confirming what I already knew: we were kin. Our first verbal interaction felt like a culmination of the ones we'd been conducting silently for months.

Dalya became my doula for the birth of my second daughter. She was by my side during my beautiful day-long labor at our house; when, after arriving at the hospital after fourteen hours of contractions, I learned that I was only three centimeters dilated and they tried to send me home. I insisted on immediate admittance and a prompt C-section, something I had been hoping to avoid up until that moment, and I know it was her presence that enabled me to feel sure in my decision. Words rarely fail me, but I don't have much more to offer than this: our bodies had been in conversation for a long time—it is a pure, animal connection, maybe even spiritual, one that doesn't totally make sense in daily life. Dalya and I have mutual friends, I'm sure we'd have fun barbecuing or playing board games, but our relationship exists on a different plane.

I've developed relationships with a handful of other regulars. I think of them as a kind of family. We chat after class, and surprisingly intimate things sometimes tumble out. When we part, I tell them I love them, only wondering later during the drive home if that was a weird thing to do, if it is true. I never see these people outside of our dance space, but here we have been so open and vulnerable, shared so much and so many bodily fluids, how could it not be true? Yes, even if they think it's strange, it's okay, I decide. I do love them.

The pandemic made in-person Dance Church impossible for over eighteen months. If I ever doubted my love for my dance fam, being away from them made it clear. I missed them like a limb that had been cut off, in a way that it took me months to admit. These "casual friendships" are actually anything but—they are part of the fabric of my life, apart from my family, my responsibilities. These are people who know another side of me, a version of me, a me that has always existed. Through dance, my body has forged ties—ones not defined by the traditional notions of friendship—that are nonetheless very real.

IN WESTERN CULTURE THE RATIONAL, well-contained mind is considered superior to the messy, physical body. The mature, developed psyche—critical, moral, intelligent—takes precedence over the runny nose, flailing arms, and flatulent viscera that it sits above. The body is seen as primitive compared to the highly complex brain. But as research and a deeper understanding of the human nervous system make their way into the psychological establishment, as well as mainstream consciousness, this paradigm is undergoing a major overhaul.

As I write this, Dr. Bessel van der Kolk's *The Body Keeps the Score: Brain, Mind, and Body in the Healing of Trauma,* is a *New*

York Times bestseller for its sixty-sixth consecutive week. Van der Kolk's work explicates not only how trauma rewires brains *and* bodies, but also how healing must happen on both psychological and somatic fronts. Recovery cannot be achieved through top-down processing alone. According to van der Kolk, it must also occur from the "bottom up, by allowing the body to have experiences that deeply and viscerally contradict the helplessness, rage, or collapse" that traumatized people remain mired in.[5] Our bodies not only hold invaluable knowledge, they transfer that knowledge to inform our mental and emotional health. The feelings of safety, closeness, and agency that we require early in life are given—or denied—to us by caregivers. Mothering is skilled labor because it cultivates this bodily knowledge that informs how we show up in the world throughout our lives.

In her book *Bodyfulness*, somatic counselor and psychotherapist Dr. Christine Caldwell argues that the basic physical functions that precede intricate thoughts do so because they are just as important to who we are. Caldwell's term *bodyfulness*, a way of inhabiting our bodies and our minds, is defined by accepting moving as being of equal value to thinking. We are closer to living as our full selves when we appreciate both taking action and pausing to consider, when we create as much as we think. We develop a strong sense of body/mind identity when, Caldwell writes, "we return to our bilingual nature and are able to be comfortable with listening to both verbal and nonverbal language systems, both as we listen to our own bodies and as we relate to the bodies of others."[6]

This idea of *returning* strikes me; after all, we aren't born with verbal language. We are born with an overwhelming capacity for sensation—emerging from the floating dark of the womb into a world of light and gravity, touch and sound. We don't lack the ability to feel, to sense, to directly experience the world. Just ask any screeching newborn. We grow rapidly in the first few years of life. Our powers of sensation never go away, only fade into the background as we gain language, the ability to tell a story, enter a world that is mediated rather than directly felt. Sensual perceptions, quickly processed by our brain, become words and thoughts to be comprehended and expressed.

But there is a limit to verbal language. There is a limit to what I can explain to my children. At some point, I just have to let them experience it. My natural tendency is to explain away, to overcompensate for how I was raised. But if I can help my daughters attune to their bodies, eventually I won't have to explain so much. My hope is that I will have prepared them to trust what they feel and know in their gut, their bones.

Throughout childhood our bodies—all that constant sensory input—impact our ability to emotionally regulate in critical ways. Part of the undeniable power of caregiving is that if we don't have someone to help us when we are overwhelmed—screaming and crying in a flood of bottom-up processing—someone to validate our feelings and affirm that we can work through them, then we learn dysfunctional ways of coping. These unhealthy adaptations can have lifelong consequences. Caregiving and mothering shape the emotional expression and resilience of the next generation of adults.

How we move together, how we sit, express, and share—these are openings to envision community as we want it to be. Sweaty and half-clothed with music; uniformed and shin-guarded and making generous passes—however it looks, it's about being free and uninhibited and working as one, creating shared space safes, free of shame. Playing with kids makes it clear that moving and being in physical collaboration transcends winning and losing. Our time together in one another's physical presence is an opportunity to create and inhabit, even if just for ninety minutes, the world we want to live in. When we are denied that connection, our mental health and ability to come together suffer.

We can have rules and time limits and shared agreements in our activities, but pleasure without a specific goal lets us access the deeper, undervalued parts of us—inefficient and sloppy, maybe, but also generous, fun-loving, carefree. Ligaya dances her way through cleaning up her toys, gets distracted by a shiny object, so often that you may have to remind her to stay on task, or accept that picking up six toys will take twenty minutes. Every time I snap at her to hurry up, which is more often than I'd like to admit, I try to also consider that I am stifling some part of her in favor of following an obligation to my schedule. And for what? So she can brush her teeth at 8:01 instead of 8:09 p.m.?

"The rhetoric of efficiency . . . suggests that what cannot be quantified cannot be of value," writes Rebecca Solnit. "That that vast array of pleasure which fall into the category of doing nothing in particular, of woolgathering, cloud-gazing, wandering, window-shopping, are nothing but voids to be filled by something more definite, more productive, or faster paced."[7]

IN 2019, EXERCISE REVENUE IN the United States totaled almost $35 billion, the largest share of the global industry.[8] In a pitch to investors, the CEO of Peloton stated that the company "sells happiness."[9] Happiness, apparently, costs $1,895 dollars, plus $39 for each additional month. What happened to spontaneous moments of joy? The free time to find yourself unexpectedly delighted? We extend the American ideals of productivity and efficiency to our off-hours. When movement becomes a means to an end, not something that might take us to an unexpected place, we lose touch with the wilder, surprising parts of ourselves.

Divisions of race and class leave many of us without access to conventional ideas of health and fitness. If you are working multiple jobs, it's harder to find time to go to the gym, a membership that costs money. Childcare providers, many of them mothers of color, chase someone else's children all day, then return and do the same for their own. Look: I work from home, my days relatively unstructured, my desire for movement strong, and yet I still struggle to make time to go for a walk, to get to a dance class, because I think I should be working. I often tie activity to something practical—walk to the produce stand, do a few loops at the park after I take Noli to school. I would tell any of my friends to do activities just for themselves, but I can't even get my ass out of my chair for myself?

"A muscle that isn't exercised will lose strength and there-fore its ability to move efficiently," writes Caldwell. "The body truly operates on a 'use it or lose it' principle."[10] We *need* to move. What do we lose when we are denied the full opportunity to do that?

It's hard to find the time to play, and harder, too, when the picture of health has always seemed out of reach. I've never seen myself, brown and short and thick, presented as an ideal of anything. Popular notions of health can be harm-ful to those of us who are excluded, who feel they could never meet such standards. These messages reach us at an early age and interfere with our ability to explore our relationship to our physical selves, without the influence of society and commerce.

For disabled folks, the emphasis on exercise can be emo-tionally and physically damaging. Looking at things through the lens of disability justice can help us expand our idea of what health and movement is. Piepzna-Samarasinha calls the knowledge disabled people navigate the world with "Crip Emotional Intelligence." When it comes to exercise, intel-ligence is understanding that "if you spent the day on the couch—because there is no way of exercising that doesn't cause pain, or because you can't move much, or because you just want to—that's just fine." It's our responsibility to not shame anyone for being still "in a world where com-pleting the Ironman or going to Zumba is shoved down ev-eryone's throats with no understanding of how 'health' can hurt."[11]

A competitive approach to movement and sports can be a

positive factor in a child's development, teaching them how to collaborate with others, to push themselves to do things they doubted themselves capable of, or to deal with loss and victory gracefully. Since elementary school, my two nieces and nephew have participated in private club soccer teams, with rigorous practice and workout sessions, plus additional skills clinics. They travel to the far reaches of the area, as well as to different states, for games and tournaments. It's a significant investment of time and money, which my brother and sister-in-law, who both work full-time, certainly feel. I've heard them say that soccer might be a way get scholarships that could guarantee their kids' college educations.

Culture writer Anne Helen Petersen argues that the professionalization of kids' sports—meaning precisely the high-stakes competition involving coaching, extra training, private leagues, travel, uniforms, and scholarship talk that's happening in my family—warps what is beneficial about these activities. "It sucks the joy from the thing," she writes, reinforcing the idea that the "ultimate goal of any of that activity is not fun or bonding or even the play itself, but a foothold, any foothold, in the scramble towards career and financial stability."[12] I share her skepticism, yet I know my nieces and nephew genuinely love what they are doing. My younger niece, who experienced some serious health issues over the last year, found her greatest hope and comfort in her teammates and friends. Talking to the three of them, I know that in soccer they are actively challenging themselves—to get better, yes, but also to be satisfied, even in loss, by how they played, how they showed up.

CHILDREN NATURALLY CRAVE ACTIVITY, and we indulge their impulses daily. The playground is among the most important locations of childhood. As we get older, society dictates that we be still for long periods of time, whether that's in school or at the office. Work often involves denying the needs of our bodies. Adults are expected to spend eight hours (or more) a day at desks or on job sites, using our bodies in service of someone else.

"How have [chairs] become so fundamental that we take their presence for granted?" design historian Galen Cranz asks in her book *The Chair: Rethinking Culture, Body, and Design*.[13] It's an important question, since a growing body of research shows that prolonged sitting is actually terrible for our long-term health. Sitting for substantial stretches each day—for weeks, months, and years of your life—can pinch nerves, limit circulation, weaken core muscles, tighten hip flexors, create varicose veins, and cause back pain. Yet we still do it, forcing people to sit at schools, at offices, in waiting rooms, and in drivers' seats.

Historically speaking, we sit in chairs because back in ancient Egypt and parts of Europe, leaders wanted a way to distinguish themselves from common people who squatted and sat on low stools. Thrones were created to set some bodies higher and apart from others, and the chair is the legacy of this power flex. It's even seeped into our language, as being the chair of a department or sitting in a director's chair indicates you hold a position of authority.[14] As Cranz writes, "Biology, physiology, and anatomy have less to do with our chairs than pharaohs, kings, and executives."[15]

Instead of thinking how we might restructure days spent on our asses and at desks, we sell people saddle stools, kneeling chairs, and pedal desks—our imagination and dollars spent on staying in essentially the same places and positions. When we finally get away from our seats to enjoy some free time, we focus less on unstructured movement and play and on their replacements exercise and fitness, so much of which has been commodified.

Day in and day out—at recess, from the moment they wake up, race to our beds to jump on us, to the moment they dive into bed—children show us ways to venture back into play, the instinct-driven movement directed by the body. We might not be able to follow their lead—we who wake and immediately check our email, start brewing coffee, set the morning routine in motion. But maybe the least we could do is try to get out of their way.

IN THE 2017 FILM *MR. GAGA*, the Israeli choreographer and dancer Ohad Naharin—broad-shouldered, muscular, lionly, decidedly *intense*—proclaims that no one, regardless of their dance ability, can't be connected to physical sensation. "There is no one that isn't capable of understanding slow-fast, thick-thin," Naharin says. "There is no one that isn't capable of connecting effort and pleasure. There is almost no one that isn't able to listen to music and feel a groove."[16]

For nearly three decades Naharin was the artistic director and choreographer of Batsheva Dance Company in Tel Aviv. Soon after taking the helm at Batsheva in 1990, Naharin began developing his own movement language, which he called Gaga. Gaga started with a few words or phrases, but from there dancers moved according to what those words stirred inside of them. They were instructed to simply make the movement their bodies wanted to make. While words are the starting point, Gaga doesn't privilege the verbal lexicon. In fact, Naharin says that Gaga is an effort to teach people "how to listen to the body before you tell it what to do."

After seeing Gaga in action, non-dancer Batsheva employees wanted to participate. So Naharin began teaching Gaga People classes, open to anyone. These classes are now taught across four continents, and students include adults and children, people with developmental disabilities, and people in wheelchairs. In the film *Mr. Gaga*, Naharin, in jeans and a baseball cap, leads class: there's an older woman in a Pink Floyd T-shirt and a red velvet scrunchie, a woman with a baby strapped to her. In another scene, Batsheva dancers lead a class for disabled children. One holds a child in his arms, allowing them to experience movement together.

In 2019, at a Monday morning Gaga People class at Mark Morris Dance Center in Brooklyn, I tried to discover how to listen to my body without telling it what to do. To find out what my body knows, what exists in me that I'm not yet aware of. A lithe dancer with warm brown skin and an Israeli accent, wearing shredded pants and T-shirt, leads class.

"Open up space," he declares at the beginning of class. "Feel the skin of your feet. Feel where they touch the floor, feel where they can lead to movement and feeling up and down the spine." This I can do. "Break open the box of your chest," he then tells us and, for a moment, I panic. This will require some effort.

The first few minutes are difficult. Mentally noisy. I look around the room and my thoughts begin racing: *Is everyone here a professional dancer? Why is everyone here a professional dancer? I can't believe I didn't wear my contacts. I'm already sweating. Look, here's a senior citizen—surely I can do this better than her, right? Wow, ageist. She's probably a retired dancer who comes to every class. Hold up, there are only three other people of color in this room.*

I close my eyes and take a few deep breaths. Eventually, I stop thinking, let go of as much self-consciousness as I can in the moment. I realize I am relying on movements I prefer to make, so I try to let go of those too. Standing, we are told to "fall upward," and I surprise myself by doing this slowly, like when you trip on the sidewalk and are aware that you are going down but cannot stop it. Soon we are on the floor, limbs extended, trembling. We are moving across the room backward, protons in a particle accelerator. We should all be crashing into each other, but miraculously we are not; we've formed a single, chaotic beam of energy. It's as though a safety net has formed around each of us, woven of our own attention.

Afterward, I am exhausted. I feel like I've poked my finger into a gooey, slime-green, weird-ass part of myself that resides somewhere between my diaphragm and my bowels, maybe my jejunum. I want to keep poking and see what emerges.

THE HUMAN BODY THRIVES WITHIN a particular set of ideal conditions: core body temperature of 98.6 degrees Fahrenheit, a blood pH factor of 7.40, blood sugar concentration at 90 milligrams per deciliter, a mean arterial pressure of 93 mm Hg, and a circulating blood volume of five liters. But we live in a world filled with industrial air-conditioning, drastic temperature changes, other people's germs, and many different types of food and drink. Daily life floods our bodies with stimuli that affect all these levels, sometimes dramatically. Our bodies are always engaged in moment-to-moment adjustments to keep us at biological equanimity. This state of being and regulation is called homeostasis.

In Latin, *homeo* means "the same" and *stasis* "standing still." The term implies fixedness and inactivity, but what we've learned about bodies is that they are never still. They are in constant motion at the most basic, cellular level. Our biological systems are perpetually in flux, adapting and adjusting in dynamic equilibrium. Movement is the natural state of the human body.

Caldwell emphasizes that we exist in a continuous oscillation, going back and forth and back and forth between various states. Our organs and tissues—think of your heart expanding and contracting, your breath going in and out, your muscles tensing and relaxing, and the ionic gates of your cells opening and closing, allowing chemicals to pass through—are always moving, whether it's in and out, back and forth, right and left, up and down.[17] We sometimes find ourselves in memorable, extreme states of activation—fight or flight—but we don't spend the majority of our lives there. Even when we are healthy, our body is never resting. It is navigating a vast middle ground, working to keep us there, in order to move forward through life.

PLAY IS DEFINED AS ACTIVITY done for fun or enjoyment. But what about: doing something for no real reason other than you want to try, to see how it feels, because it's what your body is telling you to do?

I love to see my children play, the way they get in the zone. They'll run through twenty-two uninterrupted cycles of down the slide and up the ladder. They direct all their focus into setting up a stuffy party, collecting every plush animal from all corners of the house, arranging them just so, and completing the scene with a collection of garbage treasures specially chosen for the event: a dark purple colored pencil, blue marble, headlamp, mini flashlight, produce twist tie, and green truck. I love the way one will spend the entire half hour at the park running to and fro, gathering sticks, rocks, and pinecones. When they are in this place, they are rapt, wholly absorbed—and never seem more like themselves.

At seven, my oldest has never shown any interest in organized team sports. My father once commented that she wasn't very athletic, and I took great offense. She loves being active, but what she enjoys most—hiking, skiing, kayaking (all sports her father loves too)—don't align with ways my family thinks about athleticism. I'll be honest: I enjoy the fact that her preferences aren't competitive sports, that they're immersive pursuits, ones that provide a chance to be outside, in nature. I know she likes the feeling of the wind whipping through her hair, and I like that these activities lend themselves less to quantifying maximum cardio benefits and more to feeling strong in her body.

Play equals world building, imaginative and real. I see my daughters and their friends building worlds the way they want them to be, with multiple truths, where logic and time and reason don't rule over everything. Yes, they toss, dribble, catch, and kick balls, but more often they climb and jump and run and dance. They drape their bodies over each other's, over hard and soft surfaces at odd angles. They fold themselves into nonsensical positions only children can achieve, limbs rubbery and akimbo. Inspired by *Avatar: The Last Airbender,* Noli and Ruth imagine that they can direct the elements of air, water, earth, and fire with their hands. They spend hours "training"—essentially fighting, wrestling, rolling around, and engaging in good-natured hand-to-hand and leg-to-leg combat. Their bodies are different sizes, as are their appetites for competition. They are learning and establishing their physical boundaries. We grown-ups watch as they test their strength on each other, feel their power—as well as the dominance they could have—then modulate and pull back here and there so they can keep going. They listen and attune to each other instinctively. Watching them, I realize that young children often get to know and understand each other through physical and imaginative play, not words and conversation.

I know unequivocally that this type of communication doesn't go away in adulthood. Bodies talk. I think of my

Dance Church family—new mothers, librarians fighting for a union contract, nonbinary architects, Postal Service workers, medicinal plant witches—who are my clan, one set of supportive strands in a social web that I am lucky to have. No matter the stage of life, movement—playful and free—helps us learn and grow.

What if every child believed that being "good" at a sport or activity—football, badminton, or ballet; break dancing, skateboarding, or curling; fencing, jumping rope, or juggling—means that you enjoy doing it? How might this expand our understanding of sport, movement, exercise, health? We can help them develop this perspective. It might sound far-fetched, but movement is crucial to how we become people and how we continue to evolve. If we can teach our children—who soon enough will be our adolescents, teenagers, young adults, grown-ups, middle-agers, senior citizens, our future—to continue to play, what new forms of pleasure and expression might they discover?

We encourage our children to speak their minds. Let's tell them, too, to always speak their bodies.

8

MOTHERING FOR PLEASURE

I didn't know what my clitoris was until I was fourteen years old, and even then I didn't know it by name, only by touch. I found it late at night on the couch, warm under a blanket, in the dark watching *120 Minutes* on MTV. I didn't know what was happening to me, to my body, or what to call any of it— only that it felt good and I was more and more interested in making myself feel good in this particular way. I got my first boyfriend around this time; we were on the speech and debate team together. We spent a lot of time talking about books. Making out with him in his gray Jetta, or just holding his hand, made parts of me that I couldn't name feel immensely warm, made my body glow incandescent in the dark empty lots where we parked. I wanted that feeling all the time, I wanted him instinctually—but in ways I didn't fully understand. No one had talked to me about this stuff. How it would feel. How I would want to spend hours exploring our bodies and these sensations, to rollick and discover what felt unbelievably, almost intolerably good.

We never had sex. Or at least the penetrative penis-in-vagina version we are taught is the standard definition of sex. We were dorky and young and innocent, and I think we figured we'd probably get there eventually, but never actually did. We did a lot of everything else—I remember rug burns on my knees, riding his left leg, my crotch grinding into his ankle and shin as I moved up and down, as he lay back on the couch. I'd hold his penis in my hand or my mouth and we'd both writhe in pleasure—separate, individual, given with generosity by the other, experienced first together. We knew we were on that knife's edge of too young to get it but old enough to taste it, and we held each other there.

I'm startled by how nostalgic I sometimes get for this relationship. I barely remember any details of him as a person. But I can recall that particular time when I could kiss and touch someone for hours and be so lost in the sensations that it was enough to satisfy me. That I might become part of an elastic, malleable *us* and swim around in our puddle forever. I don't know why we broke up, nothing dramatic, kid stuff. I do know I got another boyfriend fairly quickly, and soon after that started having sex. By that point I felt experienced, grown up.

Once I started having penis-in-vagina sex, it was hard *not* to have it every time I hooked up with anyone. You could spend a long time making out, but the destination always seemed to be penetrative sex. And because I didn't fully understand the workings of my body—how much time it can

take to orgasm and what kind of stimulation, internal, external, emotional that I preferred—the default goal of sex was
male climax. And, of course, I wanted to give that, to think of
myself as someone attractive and competent enough to give
that.

"I UNDERSTOOD BEFORE I STARTED having sex what
it meant for a guy to finish," an eighteen-year-old female recounts in Peggy Orenstein's *Girls & Sex*. "But I had no idea
what it meant for a girl. Honestly? I still don't know. It's never
addressed. So I've gone into it all without really understanding myself."[1]

I can relate, and I hate that. I don't believe I'm angry with
any of the young men I had sex with—looking back, it's
pretty clear none of us knew what we were doing—but I am
angry at the culture that left us with so many questions and
silence, nothing to fill it in with but scripts built on male entitlement, dominance, conquest, penetration. Once you start
following that storyline, it's the default road to go down, the
path of least resistance. It seemed rare to find a partner who
knew how to center sex on both of us, make it something
collaborative.

It's the fundamental lack of self-knowledge that I share
with this anonymous eighteen-year-old that upsets me most.
Without a sense of yourself, personal bodily knowledge, all
sexual activity will be inherently, at least in part, opaque and
disembodied. The opposite of intimate. That many people

feel this way is an indictment of a poor sex education system and conversations still dominated by shame and secrecy.

"Whereas males' puberty is characterized by ejaculation, masturbation, and the emergence of a near-unstoppable sex drive, females' is defined by . . . periods. And the possibility of unwanted pregnancy," writes Orenstein. "Where is the discussion of girls' sexual development? When do we talk to girls about desire and pleasure? When do we explain the miraculous nuances of their anatomy? When do we address exploration, self-knowledge?"[2]

All I really remember about eighth-grade sex education, taught by football coach John Wylie, a large man with a mustache and a penchant for gym shorts, goes like this: erections, ejaculation, menstruation, pregnancy, STDs. The talk I got from my parents was not even about sex, exactly: it was that my virginity was a beautiful gift from God—a precious flower—that, no matter who asks for it, I should give to just one person. My husband. I don't think we ever talked about sex before or after that.

Male physical satisfaction is presented as inevitable, while female pleasure is secondary, optional. Sex education classes tend to stick to female internal parts—the uterus, ovaries, fallopian tubes, vagina. It skips over the external, which is significant: vulva, labia, and clitoris. There's also the case of the missing internal clitoris, which wraps around the vagina and—this I definitely did not know until maybe ten years ago—is made of the same spongy erectile tissue as the penis, and also becomes engorged when aroused. It is the only human organ designed solely for pleasure. To not teach this female anatomy is, as Orenstein says, the "psychological equivalent of a clitoridectomy."

Our entire country is in on the clitoridectomy.

Only eighteen states in America currently require sex education to be medically accurate, according to a 2021 overview of state policies on Sex and HIV Education compiled by the Guttmacher Institute. Just nine states require consent to be covered as an element of sexual activity. And thirty-six states, along with the District of Columbia, give parents the option to remove their child from sex ed instruction. Additionally, nearly all institutional sex ed is prevention-based.[3]

"Plenty of young people told us that they had had sex education, but that it was taught by a teacher who was mortified to be teaching it, or whose message was one of fear: of pregnancy, of sexually transmitted infections, of all the terrible things that sex could bring into their lives," write Jennifer Hirsch and Shamus Khan, authors of *Sexual Citizens: A Landmark Study of Sex, Power, and Assault on Campus.*

"Whether from school-based sex education, from their families, or from their religious upbringing, many students we spoke with had absorbed the lesson that sex was potentially terrible and most certainly dangerous."[4]

Caretakers have the privilege and responsibility of creating and modeling spaces of safety. These physical environments can look very different from each other. They can be challenging, stimulating, surprising, or soothing, but if they do not provide a felt sense of security, a child will always feel vulnerable or under threat, unable to truly connect with others.

A hypervigilant child grows into an anxious adult, one less able to form secure attachments. And without those healthy, affectionate bonds they will be less able to form the relationships necessary for survival.

What is at stake when our understanding of sex is so limited and lacking? A culture where sexual assault is common, as Hirsch and Khan's work makes clear. Also: a country where reproductive rights, seen almost entirely as a "women's issue," are heavily restricted and controlled, where bodily autonomy can never be taken for granted.

As I write, restrictive abortion bans and punitory reproductive health bills are making their way through numerous state legislatures. Lawmakers attempting to limit people's ability to access basic health care reveal their embarrassing ignorance of basic female anatomy. Take Ohio state representative John Becker, whose proposed bill to prohibit insurance companies from covering abortion states that in the case of an ectopic pregnancy—a potentially lethal situation for a person, where a fertilized egg attaches somewhere other than inside the uterus—"Insurance companies would be permitted to cover a procedure to 'reimplant the fertilized ovum into the pregnant woman's uterus.'" Such a procedure does not exist. Then there's Missouri state representative Todd Akin, who claimed that a person who is raped cannot get pregnant because "the female body has ways to try to shut that whole thing down."[5]

In this warped vision, men remain trapped in a version of masculinity and sexuality that only allows for expertise (real or imagined) and control, but not discovery, vulnerability, or wonder. The gender binary punishes all genders.

In America, controlling people's reproductive lives is a power play—it means deciding who is worthy of having a family, perpetuating both wealth and poverty through children. An important function of sex is reproduction, yes, but it is also about feeling amazing! If we don't talk about sex through this lens, it reduces the options to all or nothing, preventive or indulgent. Hirsch and Khan note that many of the college students they spoke with were unable to answer, for themselves, the question of "What is sex for?" (For the record, I believe it is for pleasure and connection—and if those two things are not present, it's not sex, but something else.)

We are overdue for a reimagining and revisioning of sex education. Absent of this, though, it falls on parents and caregivers to get a message to children first—before they receive medically inaccurate information or a mirthless view of sex.

WILL AND I STARTED TALKING to each of our daughters about sex when they were around three years old. When I say "sex," I mostly mean anatomy and a dash of body autonomy—how touching their clitoris, which is just for them, is great and feels good. We're talking the basics. Mostly I just want them to know that we will always talk about it with them, and that they can ask questions.

So far, with our younger daughter, these talks have manifested in strong vulvar pride and a comic disbelief that her daddy only has a penis, not a vagina. With our older child, questions came almost immediately—most likely because when she was three, I was pregnant with her younger sister,

so the evidence of sex, at least as a biological process of reproduction, was always present.

One evening late in my second pregnancy, as I waddled
through our hallway, Will was putting Noli to bed. Suddenly
he found himself receiving a brain dump of questions, stray
thoughts from the past day or week that, instead of just floating downstream, got caught in little eddies and swirls of her
mind, spat out just before shutting it down.

"Daddy, you put your penis in Mama's vagina?" she asks.

"Yes."

"Daddy, when you put your penis in Mama's vagina, do you
do it lying down or like on the side?"

A beat. Then, "Yes."

I admire Will's ability to let the silence stand, to not rush
to fill it. I'm one of those parents who want to talk to their
kids about everything, in part because I feel like my parents
barely talked to me about all the things I wished they had. At
the dinner table, when questions get asked, one of my biggest challenges is keeping my explanations of things to under
thirty seconds, when a child's attention span fizzles out and
I'm left talking about empire or the social safety net while
both girls have moved on to biting apple slices into the shape
of a boat or a moon or a butt.

"Well . . . ," I start on a grand exhale, and I see all the
members of my family settle into their chairs a bit, a sign that
they are all thinking, "here she goes again . . ."

I would rather err on the side of too much information,
which is all I ever want, than not enough. But it's a process,
learning to hold back, dropping one or two important bits of

knowledge, letting that stew in their little brains. It's hard to have faith that my kids will always want to talk to me, something I didn't want to do with my parents for probably twelve years straight, that these are conversations we might be having over our lifetime together.

Sometimes I have to take a deep breath and remember what Will tells me as he rolls his eyes: "Not every moment has to be teachable."

AFTER A SNOWSTORM, WE GO into the yard and build a snowman in the field next to our house with a carrot nose and a wool fedora. Our twentysomething neighbors go out and build a five-foot sculpture of an erect penis that is fully visible to both children at all times from our living room window. When they ask us what it is, we tell them. They have no follow-up questions.

The next day, Noli's best friend is over and comments on the sculpture. "What is it?" I hear Ruth ask, as I eavesdrop from the living room.

"Oh, it's a penis," Noli replies.

"A penis??"

"Yeah, but it's standing up, not the lying down kind like my daddy's," Noli says.

THE FIRST STEP TO GETTING down is figuring out what sex even means to you, anyway.

There is no script, no formula, and no defining act. Just you, your partner, and all the things that make your bodies feel good. You can define sex however you want! And you can change that definition at any time!

It's hard to imagine being able to articulate your boundaries, wants, desires, or concerns with anyone if you haven't really communicated it to yourself.[6]

This advice, applicable to all people, comes from A. Andrews's illustrated book *A Quick & Easy Guide to Disabled Sex*. I found it remarkably helpful, refreshing, and true to the confusing and sometimes embarrassing condition of having a body and having feelings. When you bring queer and crip sex into the conversation, it's clear just how limited our understanding—and the lessons we teach—about sex really are. In learning about disability and disability justice, I've found a helpful way of approaching sex—both for my children and for myself.

Here, too, the crip emotional intelligence that Piepzna-Samarasinha writes about is invaluable. It is "understanding there are a million ways to be sexual (if one is sexual) and some of them live in phones, don't ever involve genitals, happen once a year," they explain. "[It's] understanding that all movement is movement, and counts, including when someone can only move three fingers and part of their forehead. All sex is sex."[7]

ONE OF THE MOST INFLUENTIAL and enduring forces of Spanish colonialism in the Philippines is Catholicism. The majority of Filipinos and Filipinx Americans are Catholic, so they are taught that sex outside of marriage is wrong, birth control should not be used, abortion is a sin.

Meanwhile, precolonial Indigenous views of sex and sexuality went more like this: sexual pleasure was a mutual goal, as much about female satisfaction as male. According to historian Luis Francia, in Indigenous Filipino cultures "virginity was neither prized nor desirable, and polygamy was accepted—both of which practices the zealously Catholic Spanish attempted to and did for the most part wipe out." Coming from a patriarchal culture of machismo, Spanish conquistadors found sexually independent women disturbing and intolerable.[8]

My daughters are young, and nature is one of the primary lenses through which we see and process the world. The dark purple of Japanese maples; the chick-a-dee chick-a-dee sounds of the black-capped chickadees; the fat rabbits and the baby rabbits that live in the field next to our house; the yellow jackets that sting us and the bumblebees that do not; the riot of fuchsia rhododendrons that mark each spring. They all contribute to how we talk about skin color and pigmentation, body shapes, and every living thing's inherent value. The beauty in variety, and nature's absolute insistence on it at all levels. And so, too, with sex.

Nature is queer and abundant. It is homosexual and trans, it is communal and affectionate. Though we may not find these stories widely in children's books, the animals my daughters are taken with, it turns out, are quite taken with rump bumping, same-sex diddling, licking, and nuzzling. Male giraffes love to neck and arouse each other; female bonobos like to rub clits. For fun, a male Amazonian river dolphin called a boto will insert his penis into another male's blowhole (on its head! I know Ligaya will really get a kick out of this). Male orangutans sometimes retract their penis into their body to form a space for other males to penetrate with their penis. Fingers in the butt, tail fins into genital slits, and please let's not forget the spinner dolphins, who engage in mutual sessions of caressing and arousing activities, both same-sex and opposite-sex, that zoologists have brilliantly termed "wuzzling."[9] Such creativity and obvious prioritization of pleasure makes the narrow choices for sexual expression that I see in mainstream human culture all the more disappointing.

I'm not suggesting that we return to precolonial Filipino sex (though I am open to it) or that we all wuzzle like spinner dolphins, but the more I discover, the more sex feels freer, more expansive. These ideas exist in people and animals, naturally, but they have been erased. We have been removed from who we are, and the possibilities of how we can manifest ourselves.

How much of my life is unlearning what I thought I knew about sex, what scraps I gathered and blended with cultural messaging and my desire to be sexual, liberated, powerful? How many times have I performed some idea of "sexy," not knowing what I actually thought that looked like? How many years did I live under the idea that being powerful and "sexy" meant approaching sex like a man, wanting to dominate, and taking control before realizing that's not actually what I want, nor an accurate representation of my sexuality?

My friend tells me a story about a fight she had with her

husband. They have different sex drives, but had fallen into a pattern of him, sometimes desperately, asking for sex and her, sometimes coldly, turning him down, which are not the positions either of them wants to be in. What came out of their discussion, she told me, was a wave of anger, a flushing out of bad feelings and memories, disgust at every blow job she'd reluctantly given. "When you touch the back of my head when I'm going down on you," she told him, "what I feel isn't you—it's every person who's ever pushed me to do it when I didn't really want to."

It occurs to me as she is telling this story that it really isn't just about him, or even about her. She is, sadly, telling a story about what it is like to be a typical woman our age in America. How many times have we settled for bad sex when we really didn't want it, just because we didn't quite know how to get out of it, and it seemed "easier" to just do it and get it over with and get on with life?

I ASK MY HUSBAND ABOUT his first impressions of sex. His father, a former Catholic priest, was a Catholic school teacher and his first sex ed teacher. "That it's wrong, that my desires are sinful," he says.

"What helped you undo that?"

"I'm still undoing it. Every time I feel desire, a sexual want, the first thing I have to do is tell myself that it's okay, I'm entitled to it."

I stop myself from saying that I think this is maybe the saddest thing I've ever heard.

I think back on the early days of our relationship, when our knees touching under the bar sent an electric rush through me, when physicality and sex came freely and often. That connection was real, the spark that brought us together. At times I've mourned or lamented the overall decrease in sex, at times I've welcomed and felt relieved by it, but I've never worried too much—because as our relationship has grown, so have the layers and texture of our lives. Sex is just one part of how we stay connected, just as travel, parenting, cooking, bingeing *Survivor*, and nursing each other through illness have been. But I do wonder: How much of our sexual lives together have we spent playing roles we think we should play, being as much ourselves as we could be, not realizing we haven't yet gotten to who we are underneath it all? Because neither of us actually knows?

IN HIGH SCHOOL, I HAD the fortune of having one teacher I adored. She oversaw the school newspaper and was my speech and debate coach. Once, during my senior year of high school, we were in the process of picking out new poems for me to read aloud.

She came to me with a poem by Sharon Olds, the title of which I forget. For some reason, when we met and I read the poem aloud, we were in a hallway. I remember sitting on the floor in a little alcove, speaking in quiet voices. I read the poem. It was obviously about sex (which at this point in my life I was having) and death and grief. I struggled with it. I remember telling her, "I don't get it." She told me—and I remember because this was the first time in my life an adult talked to me about sex like I was an adult—that, after the loss of her husband's mother, they had found great comfort and beauty in sex. That it was a way to grieve, a way to be closer to him, the kind of physical communion that Olds was describing. I remember so clearly, amid the too cold air, the sterile cream walls, surrounded by lockers, feeling too young and out of my depth, but also grateful to her and saying, "I still don't get it." Sex had never been that for me. I was a child playing at it, had no idea that sex could be another dimension of connection and emotion. We found another poem.

I have thought about that moment in the hallway quite a few times since. Teenagers can be trusted to hear these things; they can be trusted to realize that they are not old enough to comprehend something. So why not try? I had a fair amount of sex before I ever grasped what my teacher told me that day. I didn't understand it until I was thirty-four years old.

After getting married, my husband and I left our jobs and our home to travel for a year—South America, East and West Africa, Southeast Asia. We had left Seattle in October, and in December, as we were about to travel from Argentina to Brazil, I got word that a good friend from home had suffered a brain aneurysm. She had been feeling off, tired and weak, for months. When she finally went to the doctor, the aneurysm was discovered, and they recommended immediate surgery. I learned all of this in an email from a mutual friend. Surgery didn't go well, and she emerged from it in a coma. She remained unconscious until her death, a few days after Christmas. All of this happened in a few short weeks. When

I found out that she had passed away, we were near Salvador, Bahia, and had just gotten back from a few days on a remote island. I felt so far away, in grief, but also disconnected from reality, from anything familiar, anything tangible to prove she was really gone.

And then, that night, legs tangled in our sandy sheets, it happened—it clicked, and body and brain understood what I had been told all those years ago. Sex could be a place where bodies could do what words could not. It didn't mean turning off my brain, it meant opening up another part of it. Grounding me, pulling me back into this world, giving grief a place to flow to, someone else to absorb and share it, to show me how alive I am, how dead my friend really was.

"While our need for intimacy has become paramount, the way we conceive of it has narrowed. We no longer plow the land together; today we talk," writes Esther Perel. "In our era of communication, intimacy has been redefined. No longer is it the deep knowledge and familiarity that develop over time and can be cultivated in silence. Instead, we think of intimacy primarily as a discursive process, one that involves self-disclosure, the trustful sharing of our most personal and private material—our feelings."[10]

FOR A SHORT WHILE, FOR PARITY, I demanded that I have an orgasm every time we had sex. Before his penis could enter my vagina my husband needed to put in much manual labor, external and internal. I make it sound like a job, which isn't entirely fair and it's not like he didn't enjoy the work, but it hardly felt like a joint venture. It had a way of leeching the fun from things, and when I thought an orgasm wouldn't happen, I'd get annoyed and just want to quit. We'd finish, and the first thing I'd say is that he "owed me one." I was so busy stat tracking that I lost sight of why I was having sex in the first place.

What if, instead of climaxing, the motivation was just to feel good and aroused for as long as possible? To sustain that feeling, dwell in it, push deeper. Not achieve, not be efficient, not have it come to a tidy end.

Orgasms sometimes seem like an annoying goal—another thing to achieve, an accomplishment. In middle age, after childbirth and pregnancy, after the stripping away of libido because of depression and antidepressants, the sex I like best is just about blissful sensation. Free of any expectations, any rules, any idea we've been taught, any idea we mistakenly decided twenty years ago that we wanted to embody. I want to be lost in interminable, amorphous pleasure. To just roll around and not worry about time or my body, just be in it. That's what I want now, though I suspect it will change again.

I no longer approach sex expecting clarity or understanding. Maybe I turn to it for precisely what it gives me that I cannot say or ask for? I have to listen to my body's desire for it, how it responds to my partner. Sex now, as our marriage gets older and smarter and also more tired, isn't what I thought it was. Did I even know what I thought it was?

Last summer, after four straight months of rain and quarantine, we dropped off our children with their grandparents for a few nights so we could go camping in warmer, drier

Eastern Washington. We found a primitive campsite on fish and wildlife land, on a mountainside above a small town. We set up our tent, but found ourselves, despite the mosquitoes buzzing around, lying together on a blanket in the open air. It had been a long time since we had just touched each other for a sustained period of time, without knowing almost exactly what would happen. Hours were lost on that blanket, and my skin felt fuzzy, like the polar friction between two magnets that are attracted, in relationship, though they won't quite come together. Beneath two towering trees joined by a wooden beam nailed into them—a place for hunters to hang carcasses—I got on my hands and knees. Will put his hand inside me in a way that felt urgent and searching, deeper and more crass than ever, but also lovely and idyllic right there amid the crickets chirping and ducks chatting at the nearby pond. I came, sort of, but mostly I felt like I was in a constant state of coming the whole time we were there. At some point I gestured toward his semihard dick, a vague inquiry, and he laughed—yeah it wasn't that hard, but whatever, he said, batting it with his hands, back and forth: this is what a happy dick looks like, it can still feel everything, let's go.

We converged on that trip, but something broke too: any preconceived notion of what might happen, what should happen. There was only the moment, only the universe and warmth that happened as we touched, we were swimming in it, coming up for air, diving back into it, floating on our backs, treading—did it matter, really, where we were going or where we would end up?

Eleven years into marriage, sex is where we free ourselves

from feeling like parents and caregivers, reinhabit our bodies. When we meet, I feel closer to grasping who I am sexually. It's dialogue, a give-and-take. Sometimes we just grope in the dark for minutes, maybe hours. The goal, if there even is a goal, is curiosity, sensation, openness.

It's the spirit and ethos of sex that we've been feeling our way toward for a while—as much an unlearning of what we were told as it is a deliberate movement toward. It's all the things men aren't taught to do, and many of the things I rejected as a woman to seem more powerful than I felt, because I mistakenly thought it was about power. Now we can go to new places made possible by familiarity and freedom, and it's more playful, more tender, more thrilling.

What do I want for my daughters? To be with their pleasure, to not have an idea of what it has to be, an idea to live up to. To know that self-discovery takes time and exploration and effort, and they can both do so at their own pace, because they'll be doing it for most of their lives. To know that more is possible in sex when it's done in real relationship with someone—based in respect, mutuality—even if you don't know someone that well.

I'M ABOUT TO WALK AWAY when I hear my daughter, ready to drift off, lob a few more sex questions at my husband.

"When you put your penis in Mama's vagina, do you do it in the water?"

"Sometimes yes."

"Do you do it, like, in a hotel?"

"Oh yeah, definitely."

I resist the urge to barge in and join their conversation. Instead, I relax and let go, let my weight press into the doorframe and listen—to their breathing, him stroking her hair and giving a final kiss goodnight. I let myself look forward to a future conversation when she has more questions, when I get to look her in the eyes and speak openly. I am ready.

9

MOTHERING AS NATURAL INTERDEPENDENCE

For the last three years, Noli has talked consistently about becoming a botanist. She pauses during walks to pick and assemble humble bouquets: clover flowers, tall grass going to seed, dandelions, buttercups, sweet peas. She collects rocks and oyster shells, seagrass, sticks that catch her eye, and moon snail shells. She arranges and rearranges all of them in a small patch of dirt by our house that she calls "Nature City." Her Aunt Dodo sent her a simple plastic microscope as a gift, which she immediately began using to examine pinecones and pine needles, acorns and seedpods. She is fascinated by the sticky pitch that leaks out of the cedar tree that shades our patio, which she calls "zap," and which I absolutely refuse to correct her on. This past summer, she attended one week of camp at an urban farm, where each morning they made tea with herbs from the garden. Now, when we go for walks, she hollers, "Chicory!" and tries to gather roots for some future concoction. When she has a mosquito sting that is itching her, she stoops over a plant and says, "I'll just pick some of this plantain and rub it on the bite."

Before all the botany talk, she hadn't seemed particularly interested in any one thing, at least not in the way some of her friends had taken to baseball, ballet, or Minecraft. But after camp it became clear this is a real interest, one that could benefit from some gentle encouragement. Sometime, when she was around age five, I noticed that she began seeming less like a kid, like *my* kid, and more like her specific self. There was a self-possession taking hold, a tender green stalk of confidence shooting up inside of her. Since then I've pushed myself to really see and know her, not the set of impressions of her I've been acquiring over the years. I don't want her identity to get fixed in my mind, I want it to be fluid. To follow her lead is practice at keeping my ideas of her nimble and dynamic.

Back from a special camping trip with her father, Noli vibrates with excitement as she tells me that they found and identified many sword ferns, and that she can tell them apart from other ferns because, at the base of each leaf, they are joined to the stem by a "thumb." On a walk, she takes the time to show me, and I see it: a tiny protrusion, a squat digit of green that I'd never noticed before. "Yup, there it is!" I say. I look at her in appreciation. She gives me a double thumbs-up.

Being with her is humbling. It deepens my feeling that, for much of my life, I had it ass-backwards.

As a kid, my family never went camping. I remember long road trips in our big van with graphic brown decals, stopping at rest stops, and playing "I Spy" games as we drove. And I can picture clearly, on green "Lodging" highway signs, the many bright yellow squares of the KOA logo: a red and black tent (or was it a teepee?) that was mysterious to me. Camping was just not something we did. We piled into cheap hotel rooms—sometimes on extended family road trips, six or seven kids in a room. But buying tents, camping stoves, sleeping bags, and lying on the ground just wasn't part of our definition of vacation or fun. I think of it this way: my parents are immigrants from the Philippines. Dirt floors were something they were actively trying to get away from.

I grew up believing hiking and camping were not activities for someone like me, and I resisted them. For years I thought being active in the outdoors required money, and gear. Camping. Skiing. Tennis. Golf. I saw all of these as rich white people activities that, with all the equipment required, were what white people spent their money on.

We lived in the woods of rural Pennsylvania, but the woods wasn't some special destination. It was just our backyard. When my parents had the trees behind our house felled to make a full driveway so we wouldn't have to walk up the hill to our front door, the pile of fallen hemlocks became a place I could crawl around in after school in my navy-and-green plaid Catholic school skirt and white Peter Pan blouse, an overgrown maze of my own making. Just up the hill in the woods behind our house was a large swatch of green moss, the private patch of plush carpeting where I daydreamed. But always, even after blissful hours and whole afternoons spent climbing trees and getting sap stuck to my clothing, I returned home. To a shower. A warm bed.

I was, in ways I couldn't yet see, lucky enough to take my situation for granted. To see the woods as an extension of myself, my world, our home. Starting in adolescence, my life seemed to be about getting away from everything I had known. The small town, the nearly all-white community, the seemingly limited scope. I imagined a bigger world, a densely packed world, an urban world. "We call it 'Nature'; only reluctantly / admitting ourselves to be 'Nature' too," writes poet Denise Levertov, who is buried on a hill in Seattle, where I've now lived for over twenty years.[1]

MY FIRST IMPRESSIONS OF SEATTLE were all linked to its natural beauty. The landscape is majestic. On the best days, a heaven realm: a city on the edge of salt water, as well as the shores of multiple lakes, with views of two snow-capped mountain ranges—the Cascades and Olympics—to the east and west. Here there are infinitesimal shades of gray and green. I spent many years wanting to escape the woods but had to admit that here, the evergreens, mountains, trails, and water all called in some way.

Aside from drives and walks along Lake Washington, though, I didn't really know how to engage with nature. During my early twenties my leisure activities mainly consisted of drinking whiskey and smoking cigarettes in dark bars, yelling about books, and going to music shows. Culturally, I identified more with creative types—the people I worked at an independent bookstore with, the writers at the alt-weekly where I interned. Aside from swimming in the lake, none of these people seemed to be heading out into the woods on the weekend. In this city, home of REI, outdoor leisure is also synonymous with equipment: zip-up Polartec fleece, ultralight tents, hydrating CamelBak backpacks, hiking boots, and all-terrain sandals with Vibram soles. They showcase people's financial resources as much as the time they have to be leisurely.

When I met my husband, I had a hard time imagining us together. He wore zip-off waterproof convertible pants, where the bottom half of each leg comes off to create a pair of shorts. Most weekends, he wore the same dark gray performance gear shirt with silver raglan sleeves. He loved skiing. He grew up in Colorado where, he told me, everyone skied, no matter how much money they had. I was dubious. He spoke of the importance of wicking and warned how, in the outdoors, "cotton kills." He used to rock climb, and his closet was filled with specialized lace-up climbing shoes, carabiners, and miles of rope. He owned an ice axe. He used something called a Beacon, a radio signaling device that could be used to locate a skier if they were buried under snow or in a tree well after an avalanche.

Everything about his physical body read privilege to me. And indeed his body—thin, white, healthy, athletic, male— moved through the world with a tremendous ease he took for granted. It still does. The problem was I wasn't reading him properly. Closely enough. With any kind of generosity. We met in the summer. By winter, months into dating, in love, he was heading out on mountain weekends, putting dates off so he could go skiing after work. I saw that his skis were . . . old. Dinged up. They were the same ones he'd been skiing on since he was a teenager. His poles were bent and mismatched. His winter coat (a "soft shell," I was told) smelled like mold. He never had it cleaned, never let it dry properly, just let it sit for hours in a dark closet absorbing melted snow.

For Christmas, he got me a Patagonia fleece. I worried that he was trying to turn me into someone more like him. More like other women he dated. (I didn't know anything about his exes, just that his most recent one was into Burning Man.) It's taken me years to realize that, despite how curious I am about people, however extroverted I am—my default approach is still guarded, suspicious, self-protecting. I thought he wanted to change me; he just wanted to share the things he enjoyed with me. To share himself with me.

I agreed, sometime in the middle of Seattle's interminable gray drizzly winter, to go on a hike. I had one condition: that it be a rewards-based hike, with something beautiful at the end. He pored over his guidebooks and found one—it was a little long but with moderate elevation gain, he said, totally manageable, with a waterfall at the end.

The day we went out, it was clear weather, so I wore my glasses rather than contacts. In the mountains, it was raining. I had my fleece, but I didn't own a raincoat. It started out well enough; we passed a slug the size of my hand and marveled at it. But the trail kept climbing, and it just kept getting wetter. I was trying to be a good sport and, because I am competitive by nature, I didn't want to give up. But I was miserable and becoming less interested in hiding it. Eventually we arrived at an alleged alpine lake—the fog and mist were so thick we couldn't see it. There was no sign of the waterfall and we'd already hiked all the miles I was told we'd be hiking. I yelled that this was bullshit and demanded that we turn back, and what the hell was wrong with him, couldn't he see how wet and cold and unhappy I was and that I couldn't see a fucking thing through my glasses. It was like driving in a rainstorm without windshield wipers. We turned back. I rushed ahead of him and stayed ahead the entire way down—muttering expletives, fists clenched, blowing fumes out of my nose, anything to show him how pissed off I was.

Despite that early setback, Will proved unflappable. He eased up on mentioning hiking or backpacking or camping until early summer, and this time he came prepared. He proposed a one-mile hike on the Olympic Peninsula to natural hot springs. I was skeptical, but hot springs—it was too much to resist. It would be a backpacking trip, where we would carry everything we needed: tent, sleeping bags, food. I asked if we could bring my eight-inch cast-iron skillet to cook steaks or bacon or eggs in. "Of course!" he said.

It would be years before I learned that, when backpacking, pack weight is critical and, especially on longer trips, people strive to keep their bags as light as possible. Many people don't even bring food to cook—they eat things such as peanut butter tortilla roll-ups, energy bars, and nutritional goo. Maybe the biggest gesture of love Will has ever offered me is not laughing directly in my face when I asked to carry a cast iron.

After I'd been dating Will for a couple of years, my brother, sister-in-law, and their kids came out from Pennsylvania to visit one summer. My sister-in-law was a big *Twilight* fan, so we rented a simple cabin out at La Push, where the *Twilight* books and movies are set, and decided to cook dinner out on the beach. I thought I would impress them with my (newly acquired) camping skills, starting a fire and cooking on the coals. But the beach was windy, and I struggled to get it going. After a few minutes my sister-in-law Amy took pity on me and offered to help. She got onto her knees, bent down low, and had the kindling lit almost instantaneously. I was embarrassed and impressed. I had no idea she could do that, I said.

"I grew up camping," she told me. "My family never had any money. All of our vacations were camping vacations."

As soon as the words left her mouth I felt like an idiot. Here I had seen everything about outdoor recreation from the perspective of a non-white person, but I had never considered how much financial privilege my non-white family had. And now this member of my family was handing me dinner and a lesson on a platter, a campfire-kissed envelope of aluminum foil.

OVER THE YEARS, I'VE REKINDLED and formed a new relationship with nature. In youth, my view of the world wasn't so nuanced that I could see how life in the city and

life in the woods weren't opposites. I saw it as a choice between things, needing to reject one for the other, not realizing it doesn't have to be that way. At some point during all
those seemingly endless hikes that Will took me on, I gave
in, found my rhythm, found pleasure. I walked slowly. I didn't
force anything. For so many people—immigrant, Indigenous,
folks of color—separated, often forcibly, from the land, and
essentially barred from cultivating an unmediated relationship to the earth, it's healing to return to it. To rediscover it
on your own terms.

The realization I made was so simple as to be stupid, but
transformative nonetheless: hiking is just walking. My body
was built to walk. When I start out hiking, I tend to be nervous, with an excess of energy that means I hit the trail a little hard. But over the years, I've started to relax. I tell myself
always, it's just walking. One foot in front of the other. I hear
the words of Bonancio, the Quechuan guide who led us on
an ancient Incan highway for three days, a walk that started
high in the mountains of La Paz, ending in the lush and hu-
mid jungle of the Amazon. "A tu paso," he would say to me
with a comic bow and a dramatic sweep of the arm, as though
he was laying out the whole world. *At your own pace.* Moving
at that speed, I began to see the natural world as open and
available to me—my birthright for being a human on earth.

I learned all of this so late.

Will and I have since hiked and backpacked throughout
Washington State and when traveling in other countries: the
North Cascades, the Olympic Coast, the Quilotoa Loop in Ec-
uador, the mountains of northern Luzon, through the Simien

Mountains in Ethiopia. Each time I am struck by how local guides mostly hike in flip-flops, with no special gear. Many of them smoke cigarettes as they climb thousands of feet. It's just what people do, one way of moving through the world.

I like my body in these places, places that are always there, stalwart and unbothered, but also temperamental and extreme. I'm a body, pulsing and breathing, but I'm also nothing, absorbed into a vast everything. I'm aware that my body, a miraculously complex system, is just another body. On a trip to the town of Stehekin on a remote shore of Washington's Lake Chelan, I knew how easily I could be swallowed by the frigid water, no more important than the leaves falling into it from the trees above, the fish that make it their home, or the migratory geese who found it a pleasant enough place to stop on their journey. Places like this are not necessarily where I want to live every day, but increasingly they are where I want to spend some time.

"Whenever we lose track of our own obsessions," writes Levertov, "then something tethered in us / hobbled like a donkey on its patch / of gnawed grass and thistles, breaks free." This looking outward, taking in a new place, experiencing a change in perspective might be profound, but it happens inside of us, undetectable by others. In Levertov's words, "No one discovers / just where we've been . . . /—but we have changed, a little."[2]

THERE ARE PEOPLE WHO CAN go through life without any conscious relationship with nature, just as there are people who could never imagine living without the wilderness. I think more of us exist in an in-between, and our lives and schedules jimmy us into a relationship different from the one we'd have if left to our druthers. If I never suggested going outside, I honestly believe my four-year-old, who starts every day by asking, "Can we watch TV?" would happily spend most of her time in the house. And yet, when she gets outdoors, there she is. She'll stay for hours. She wants to climb, to put her finger into holes in trees, to poke dirt and debris with sticks, gather rocks, chase squirrels. At any body of water—even a public fountain—it takes less than five minutes before she turns to me and says, "Mama, it's okay if I get naked and in the water?"

It's here, in each person, an elemental connection with nature: the feeling of cool grass between sour-smelling toes; breeze caressing a cheek; the surprising splash of salt water in the eyes when its surface is broken. It's easier to access as children, though—before adulthood, work, and responsibilities wrest us away from it. I want us to find our way back.

How might we remind ourselves, as Levertov says, that we, too, are nature? It involves a bit of ego death, of letting go, admiring growth that expands in unpredictable directions rather than forward progress. In his 1949 book *A Sand County Almanac*, Aldo Leopold proposes a Land Ethic, an ethos that "enlarges the boundaries of the community to include soils, waters, plants, and animals." Sounds easy enough, but the kicker is that the land ethic "changes the role of homo sapiens from conqueror of the land-community to plain member and citizen of it."[3] This is the part we homo sapiens have trouble with.

In her book *How to Do Nothing,* Jenny Odell offers bioregionalism as a way to help us better situate ourselves within our communities. Bioregionalism is "based on observation and recognition of what grows where, as well as an appreciation for the complex web of relationships among those actors," she writes. But more than looking and identifying, bioregionalism "suggests a way of identifying with place, weaving oneself into a region through observation of and responsibility to the local ecosystem."[4]

What we're really talking about is an approach to community that simply asks you to make the effort to learn the names of some of your (nonhuman) neighbors and remember a few details about their lives. For me the most appealing aspect of bioregionalism is that it's a way to fight the dissociative and amnesiac feelings that seem to be part of daily life in America. Here's something that happens to me often, more times a day than I'd like to admit: when I find myself experiencing a difficult thought that I'd prefer not to be having, I reach for my phone and scroll through Instagram, or play Spelling Bee, or check my email—anything to distract me from my inconvenient feelings. I feel temporarily better, but all I've done is momentarily separate me from myself and give my attention to a device that ultimately gives me nothing in return except anxiety, my same neuroses, the joyless feeling of having compared myself, and the compulsion to mindlessly keep scrolling, scrolling, scrolling.

Just outside the window above my desk is a lodgepole pine tree. This tree has lived at our house longer than we have, and I've looked at it nearly every day while writing two books, dozens of articles, and countless emails over the last eight years. I wonder which of the three previous owners of this house planted it—the pianist who had the home custom built in 1975 but only lived here for two years? The woman who lived here for twelve years but who I know nothing about? The Wongs? I didn't learn the lodgepole's name until this year, after Noli got a Pacific Coast tree guide, and I stopped to look closely at it: how its thin green needles, sharp at the tip, grow in clusters of two and have a twist to them, like naturally wavy hair or just a teeny bit like those inflatable dancing tube men outside of check-cashing places and car dealerships. I used to generically call the trees that shield our house from wind and rain "evergreens," but now I see that the lodgepole is entirely different from the Western red cedar next to it whose needles grow like scales, bundled and layered on top of each other, and whose branches droop melodramatically.

Now, when my family goes clamming on the Hood Canal, using a rake and our bare hands to dig through cold gray sand, we know the difference between the littlenecks, manilas, and varnish clams. While the littleneck is native, the thriving manilas and varnishes are technically invasive, having hitched a ride across the Pacific in the ballast water of ships carrying oyster seed from Japan. We know varnish clams are tasty but that toxins stay in their soft bodies longer, so it's best to avoid them in warmer months. Along the coast, I love the sight of abundant ocean spray, a thin-stemmed plant with bursts of creamy white flowers. Coast Salish peoples used the wood to make sewing needles, spears, and harpoons. It might look flimsy, but the wood is hard and dense and can be made stronger by holding it to fire. It reminds me of some people I know.

Whatever you call it, I've found that paying this kind of attention to living things around me counteracts the separation I feel from myself when I give my attention to things that don't really matter, or that mean far less to me. When I'm looking around, I'm indulging my curiosities, the aspects of myself that I don't yet know, that are willing to go on a long walk and get lost, that have no obvious value.

"I like walking because it is slow, and I suspect that the mind, like the feet, works at about three miles an hour," writes Rebecca Solnit. "If this is so, then modern life is moving faster than the speed of thought, or thoughtfulness."[5]

My phone, my Google calendar, my Roku television with NBA League Pass—these technologies separate us from our unoccupied thoughts and the places we might sit with them, as well as the insects, birds, and small mammals who might join us there. We often fill these spaces with addictions and compulsions—all kinds of things that make us feel shitty, that get us caught in a cycle of shittiness.

"That same relationship to the richness of place lets me partake of it, too," writes Odell. "When I worry about the bird, I am also worrying about watching all my possible selves go extinct. And when I worry that no one will see the value of these murky waters, it is also a worry that I will be stripped of my own unusable parts, my own mysteries, and my own depths."[6]

I don't just want to explore the coastal rain forest and alpine trees of the Pacific Northwest. Sometimes I want to walk slowly and languidly through a tropical place, stiflingly hot. I want to feel the humidity collide with my skin and stick to it, feel the sweat start and in seconds find myself wet with my own perspiration. Sometimes I want the fecund, almost pornographic smell of fallen jacarandas, ripening mangoes, jackfruit, and papayas.

A connection with the natural world is a fundamental value to cultures that came before us, cultures that have been colonized and suppressed, whose erasure we must insist against. Indigenous Filipinos attributed supernatural powers to elements of nature. They believed their ancestors could be absorbed back into these sources, and showed great reverence for the wind, water, and stones. "To cut down an old tree, for example, was considered sacrilege," writes Luis Francia. "Or to fail to ask permission to pass in front of an ant mound in a field was tantamount to inviting retribution (usually in the form of a mischievous trick) from the mound's resident spirit."[7]

On his memorable tour of Intramuros in Manila, the late performer, artist, and activist Carlos Celdran led people on a playful walk through the historic Spanish walled city that was the seat of colonial government. Celdran told the history you don't often hear, of the double legacy of Spanish and American colonialism and how it remains: both in the Catholic faith, which gave the country a theocracy, and now a government rooted in conservative social policy, and a culture that worships celebrity, just as American popular culture does.

What I remember most, though, was what Celdran had to say about language. There are hundreds of Indigenous languages throughout the islands, but most of them have absorbed a certain amount of Spanish and English. Filipinos will refer to a tissue, whatever brand, as a Kleenex and a camera simply as a Kodak. From the Americans, we took the language of corporations and commercialization. Everyday objects are referred to by their Spanish names: table, fork, and book are mesa, tinidor, and libro. But the Tagalog and native words that persist are those things that cannot be quantified, part of nature, part of us: wind, rain, tree, soul, spirit. Hangin, ulan, puno, kaluluwa, diwa.

These are what endure.

NOLI PLAYS "SUSHI" WITH HER school friends. They run all over the park gathering white-petaled clover flowers, sturdy plantain leaves, fat wood chips, and thin, pointy sticks. When they've gathered all their materials, they set about wrapping the "rice" and slices of wooden "fish" in dark green "seaweed," spearing them together with their rudimentary toothpicks. Then they open their sushi store: all the food is free, or you can barter with them depending on what you have. As her friend Mirai says, "What is money and what is the point anyway if we just pass it back and forth and back and forth all the time?"

"Well, yeah, it's all made up," I tell her, smiling. She gets it.

At the heart of American capitalism is the notion of scarcity. It tells us that anything and everything we desire—the products we like, the education we want for our children—is inherently scarce, in danger of disappearing. Because these private, precious commodities are so hard to come by, they demand an appropriately high price—and we should hoard as much as we can lest others take our share. Living under capitalism, says botanist Robin Wall Kimmerer, too often means "we've surrendered our values to an economic system that actively harms what we love."[8]

Rather than abide by the rules of the market economy, Kimmerer asks that we consider the gift economy, which operates from a fundamental belief in abundance, and the currency of which is gratitude. When you see everything you have or are given as a gift to be thankful for, it leaves you happier and more accountable to those around you. The object or living thing you hold in your hands does not change, but your relationship to it does. The gift economy, according to Kimmerer, gives us "exactly what we long for but cannot ever purchase: being valued for your own unique gifts, earning the regard of your neighbors for the quality of your character, not the quantity of your possessions; what you give, not what you have."[9]

As much as some of us might hope to burn down the capitalist system we operate within, we don't need to wait for revolution to incorporate principles of abundance into our lives. It is possible to create gift economies that run parallel to market economies—in fact, so many of us already do this. Dropping food off for friends, watching someone's kid for a few hours, trading some light finish carpentry for an hour of massage, growing herbs on your windowsill or vegetables in your garden. This is caretaking and it is labor. It takes work to cultivate plants, to nourish people, to tend to the home. Most of us can't afford to stop thinking about money, but if we changed our relationship to it—even ever so slightly—yes, our finances might contract, but our emotional lives might expand in ways we can't yet measure or know. The gifts of the natural world are inherently diverse, queer, adaptable, creative, and enough. And that means so are we.

I DO MY BEST TO support Noli's interests: we go on walks with field guides, identify flowers, trees, and birds. I collect pinecones for her to inspect under her various magnifying tools, help her navigate indexes and tables of contents. Her habit is supported not just by me, but by her people. On a cabin weekend I tell our friend Rachel, who works in the Portland Parks Department, that Noli seems very interested in botany. On a walk to the nearby lake, Rachel points out flowers, the way some grow in a cluster called an *umbel*, stems originating from a central point like the ribs of an umbrella. She digs out a laminated plant identification sheet from her truck and gives it to Noli as a parting gift. At first Noli refuses—it's so wonderful, how could Rachel possibly stand to part with it?—but ultimately accepts it, beaming. Weeks later, Rachel sends her a care package with waterproof nature journals and sketches of leaves from her favorite tree, the red alder.

Do I think Noli will become a botanist? Probably not . . . but who knows? I know she is developing a way of seeing, a way of being in the world, how she chooses to inhabit it. One that will develop at her own speed.

I am grateful to her. I don't know the stories of all the original dwellers of the land we occupy, and likely never will, but I see things differently now. I know that Douglas fir cones are the ones that have "mouse tails" peeking out from the scales, and that legend has it that there was once a great forest fire, and the large pines let the small creatures take shelter in their branches. I am learning because of my child, and I get to learn with her, and it all feels very miraculous. It's a subtle shift, a sacred shift, but it's everything. I move between multiple worlds—past, present, future, my daughter's hand in mine. I am finally getting to know my neighbors, to be able to name them, with care and attention, and it does change my relationship to them. I know we humans are far outnumbered, and it's a welcome feeling. We aren't so significant, but we're part of something bigger, something quite beyond us.

IN HER POEM "GENERATIONS," Lucille Clifton writes that we, homo sapiens who will eventually be dirt, must be accountable to living things other than humans:

> *if it was only*
> *you and me*
> *sharing the consequences*
> *it would be different*

it would be just
generations of men
but
this business of war
these war kinds of things
are erasing those natural
obedient generations[10]

We are making plans now, Noli and I. I checked out *Gardening with Native Plants of the Pacific Northwest* from the library and we are talking about what to put in the ground come spring. Maybe just one or two plants this year, seeing what takes, what we learn, what we can do to help them along, adding as we go.

"Parenting, like life, is heartbreak followed by reality, followed by love, followed by loneliness, followed by despair, followed by jokes, followed by exhaustion," writes Carvell Wallace. "If this is what you are experiencing, you are doing it right. If you are returning over and over again to watch the simple miracle of growth, you are doing it right."[11]

In mothering, the growth I'm attuned to is no longer limited to my daughters—it's counting the tiny mint-green pinecones dripping with sap on the neighborhood Sitka spruces; following the reemergence of wolves in the wilderness we hope to take them to one day; marking Ruth and Sunny's heights every few months on our kitchen wall in colored pencil, along with Noli and Ligaya's; keeping track of the number of orcas in our local waters; even admiring the jump shot of the middle-aged dad who improves his form in the park every morning after school drop-off, weaving his way through orange traffic cone defenders made taller by pool noodles stuffed into the cone tops.

Love is acts of attention, and I love seeing how everything around us is always moving, changing, evolving, unfurling. This growth is intertwined with our children's—what ensures them all a healthy, embodied life of curiosity, gratitude, and rootedness.

I used to reject the idea that, in mothering, there is any way to judge what we are doing as "right" or "wrong," "good" or "bad." Wallace's words—written and read at the height of that first pandemic summer, burned into my mind and body along with all the grief and raw possibility of the moment— make me rethink all of that, reimagine everything.

To commit to witnessing, to "merely" showing up: mothering, fathering, parenting, leading and following, articulating what you know and admitting what you don't, doing things well, making mistakes, getting over it all and getting on with it. How is all of this anything but unequivocally right? To be part of the humbling and heroic, the smallest details that comprise a child's big, wondrous life—that is our duty of care.

ACKNOWLEDGMENTS

To Julie Will, for steady belief in my voice and vision, particularly when the writing was impossible, and for being game to change course when I found my way back. To Yelena Gitlin-Nesbit, publicist and friend, for working so hard on my behalf and always keeping it light, keeping it real. To Emma Kupor and everyone at Harper Wave for their ongoing support of my work. To Monika Woods, who saw a writing career for me before I could, for years of caring about the contract details that I cannot even imagine thinking about.

To editors who gave me opportunities to explore a few of the many aspects of mothering: Jessica Grose, Reyhan Harmanci, Edan Lepucki, and, most of all, Jen Gann, who casually but with unnerving acumen commissioned pieces that were foundational to the eventual creation of this book. To Emily Gould, for being a generous champion of my work and for responding to my "joke" that I try to submit a sloppy 3,500-word essay as a book draft with "whynotboth.gif." To Katherine Goldstein, for sharing space and inviting me to co-host her creation *The Double Shift,* and Rachel McCarthy, who also kept me committed to telling the stories of mothers and caregivers.

To the Seattle Public Library, for free access to the many books and ideas that informed this work. To Kultura Arts, Seattle Office of Arts & Culture, MLK Labor Council, Washington State Labor Council, and Foundation for Working Families for financial support during this long, strange, and frankly often dormant season of writing.

To Jen Graves, first and best reader, forever colleague and friend.

To every Fil Am and Filipinx writer, for showing and teaching and pushing me to inhabit my body and perspective, and helping me write a book I've always wanted to write. To Laura Garbes, for sharing your brilliance, yourself, and your sources with me. To Genevieve Villamora, Melissa Miranda, and Janelle Quibuyen, for inspiration, for being who you are and cultivating creativity and kapwa in all you do—utang na loob sa Janelle, for a perfect cover.

To the people throughout my life who have mothered me in various ways and helped me find my way with words: Lisa Bates, Annick Helbig, Avi Ziv, Patty Wortham, Claire Molesworth, Regan Kelly, Eli Sanders, Joseph Bednarik, Michael Wiegers, Kathleen Richards, Imelda Maico, Guenevere Rodriguez, Monique Thiry-Zaragoza, Danielle Thiry-Zaragoza, and Len Jugo Yonzon.

To my writer friends (who are also my mom friends) for keeping faith, particularly when I could not, and making this work less lonely: Lindy West, Meaghan O'Connell, Sara Franklin, and, especially, Shruti Swamy and Lydia Kiesling.

To my therapists and my prescriptions. To my Dance Church fam for connections that transcend words. To Angie, Nicolae, Percy, and Mac White; Alex, Kevin, Vivian, and Enzo Pemoulié; Becca, Jondou, Ruth, and Sunny Chase-Chen; Heather McGhee, Cassim Shepard, and Riaz Shepard-McGhee—for being our friends and our family; for sustenance, support, and so many epic hangs.

To the entire staff of the Jose Martí Child Development Center, especially Sandra Zuniga; Miss Edith and the folks at the Rainier Community Center After School Program; and Josephine Goodwin, for quality childcare and education that make my writing possible. To Penelope Oluo, best babysitter in the world.

To Ligaya Len and Noli Jo, for a lifetime of learning and love and wonder, and the peace that comes from feeling each of your hands in mine, a peace I never knew possible. To Will Pittz, for being the only one who can hold this shit down, accepting my need to disappear into the work, holding me accountable to myself and to us, and for making this life with me every day, this life I love.

To my parents, Josefina and Archimedes Garbes, for literally everything. I write in the hopes that we might understand each other as much as we care. Salamat sa inyong pagmamahal at pagtanggap sa akin hindi man tayo magtugma sa pagiisip. Mapalad akong maging anak ninyo.

NOTES

Introduction

1. Cathy Park Hong, *Minor Feelings: An Asian American Reckoning* (New York: One World, 2020), 77.
2. Jason DeParle, *A Good Provider Is One Who Leaves: One Family and Migration in the 21st Century* (New York: Viking, 2020), 7.
3. Catherine Ceniza Choy, *Empire of Care: Nursing and Migration in Filipino American History* (Durham, NC: Duke University Press, 2003), 1.
4. C.I.A. Oronce, A.C. Adia, and N.A. Ponce, "US Health Care Relies on Filipinxs While Ignoring Their Health Needs: Disguised Disparities and the COVID-19 Pandemic," *JAMA Health Forum*, 2021;2(7):e211489, doi: 10.1001/jamahealthforum.2021.1489.
5. Usha Lee McFarling, "Nursing Ranks Are Filled with Filipino Americans. The Pandemic Is Taking an Outsized Toll on Them," *STAT*, April 28, 2020, https://www.statnews.com/2020/04/28/coronavirus-taking-outsized-toll-on-filipino-american-nurses/.
6. Alexis Pauline Gumbs, China Martens, and Mai'a Williams, eds., *Revolutionary Mothering: Love on the Front Lines* (Oakland, CA: PM Press, 2016), 9.
7. June Jordan, "The Creative Spirit: Children's Literature," reprinted in Gumbs, Martens, and Williams, eds., *Revolutionary Mothering*.
8. Audre Lorde, "Uses of the Erotic: The Erotic as Power," *Sister Outsider* (Berkeley, CA: Crossing Press, 2007), 55.
9. Ligaya Mishan, "Asian-American Cuisine's Rise, and Triumph," *New York Times Style Magazine*, November 10, 2017, https://www

.nytimes.com/2017/11/10/t-magazine/asian-american-cuisine
.html.

Chapter 1: Mothering as Survival

1. Claire Cain Miller, "When Schools Closed, Americans Turned to Their Usual Backup Plan: Mothers," *New York Times,* November 17, 2020, https://www.nytimes.com/2020/11/17/upshot/schools-closing-mothers-leaving-jobs.html.
2. Tillie Olsen, *Silences* (New York: Delacorte Press, 1978), 18–19.
3. Victoria T. Grando, "Making Do with Fewer Nurses in the United States, 1945–1965," *Image: Journal of Nursing Scholarship* 30, no. 2 (1998): 147–49.
4. Rick Barot, "The Galleons 1," *The Galleons* (Minneapolis, MN: Milkweed Editions, 2020), 3.
5. Choy, *Empire of Care,* 4.
6. Elaine Castillo, *America Is Not the Heart* (New York: Viking, 2018).
7. Ishaan Tharoor, "Manila Was Known as the 'Pearl of the Orient.' Then World War II Happened," *Washington Post,* February 19, 2015, https://www.washingtonpost.com/news/worldviews/wp/2015/02/19/manila-was-known-as-the-pearl-of-the-orient-then-world-war-ii-happened/.
8. William McKinley, "Benevolent Assimilation Proclamation," December 21, 1898. https://kahimyang.com/kauswagan/articles/1379/today-in-philippine-history-december-21-1898-president-mckinley-issued-the-benevolent-assimilation-proclamation
9. Rudyard Kipling, "The White Man's Burden," 1899. http://historymatters.gmu.edu/d/5478/
10. Warwick Andersen, *Colonial Pathologies: American Tropical Medicine, Race, and Hygiene in the Philippines* (Durham, NC: Duke University Press, 2006).
11. Choy, *Empire of Care,* 31.
12. Julia Wolfe, Jori Kandra, Lora Engdahl, and Heidi Shierholz, "Domestic Workers Chartbook: A comprehensive look at the demographics, wages, benefits, and poverty rates of the professionals who care for our family members and clean our homes,"

Economic Policy Institute, May 4, 2020, https://www.epi.org
/publication/domestic-workers-chartbook-a-comprehensive
-look-at-the-demographics-wages-benefits-and-poverty-rates-of
-the-professionals-who-care-for-our-family-members-and-clean
-our-homes.

13. *Time to Say Goodbye* podcast, "Filipino Nurses and 'Better Luck
Tomorrow,'" December 8, 2020, https://goodbye.substack.com
/p/filipino-nurses-and-better-luck-tomorrow.

14. NPR's *Code Switch* podcast, "Why Are We Here?," March 31,
2021, https://www.npr.org/transcripts/982878218; *Time to Say
Goodbye* podcast, "Filipino Nurses and 'Better Luck Tomorrow.'"

15. Miller, "When Schools Closed."

16. Sarah Ruhl, *100 Essays I Don't Have Time to Write* (New York:
Faber & Faber, 2014), 157.

17. Wolfe et al., "Domestic Workers Chartbook."

18. Ai-jen Poo, "The Work That Makes All Other Work Possible,"
TEDWomen 2018, November 2018, https://www.ted.com/talks
/ai_jen_poo_the_work_that_makes_all_other_work_possible
/transcript?language=en#t-957999.

19. Jasmine Tucker, "Women Gained 57% of Jobs Added to
the Economy in October but Still Need Almost 8 Months of
Growth at October's Level to Recover Pandemic Losses," National Women's Law Center, November 2021, https://nwlc.org
/wp-content/uploads/2021/11/October-Jobs-Day.pdf.

20. Raj Patel and Jason W. Moore, *A History of the World in Seven
Cheap Things* (Oakland, CA: University of California Press,
2017), 135.

21. Emily Peck, "Policymakers Used to Ignore Child Care. Then
Came the Pandemic," *New York Times,* May 9, 2021, https://www
.nytimes.com/2021/05/09/business/child-care-infrastructure
-biden.html.

Chapter 2: Mothering as Valuable Labor

1. Alex Tizon, "My Family's Slave," *Atlantic,* June 2017, https://
www.theatlantic.com/magazine/archive/2017/06/lolas-story
/524490/.

2. Gus Wezerek and Kristen R. Ghodsee, "Women's Unpaid Labor

Is Worth $10,900,000,000,000," *New York Times,* March 5, 2020, https://www.nytimes.com/interactive/2020/03/04/opinion/women-unpaid-labor.html.

3. Patel and Moore, *A History of the World in Seven Cheap Things,* 24.

4. Sarah Jaffe, *Work Won't Love You Back: How Devotion to Our Jobs Keeps Us Exploited, Exhausted, and Alone* (New York: Bold Type Books, 2021), 28.

5. Jaffe, 44.

6. Amy Westervelt, "Inventory of Invisible Labor: The Coronavirus Edition," accessed May 2021, https://www.amywestervelt.com/unpaid-labor-calculator.

7. Silvia Federici, *Revolution at Point Zero: Housework, Reproduction, and Feminist Struggle* (Oakland, CA: PM Press, 2012), 31.

8. Rhacel Salazar Parreñas, "Migrant Filipino Domestic Workers and the International Division of Reproductive Labor," *Gender and Society* 14, no. 4 (August 2000): 561.

9. Parreñas, "Migrant Filipino Domestic Workers," 565.

10. Parreñas, "Migrant Filipino Domestic Workers," 566–67.

11. Johnnie Tillmon, "Welfare Is a Women's Issue," *Ms.,* Spring 1972, https://msmagazine.com/2021/03/25/welfare-is-a-womens-issue-ms-magazine-spring-1972/.

12. "Combahee River Collective Statement," April 1977, reprinted in *How We Get Free: Black Feminism and the Combahee River Collective,* Keeanga-Yamahtta Taylor, ed. (Chicago, IL: Haymarket Books, 2017).

13. Deb Perelman, "In the Covid-19 Economy, You Can Have a Kid or a Job. You Can't Have Both," *New York Times,* July 2, 2020, https://www.nytimes.com/2020/07/02/business/covid-economy-parents-kids-career-homeschooling.html.

14. Federici, *Revolution at Point Zero,* 18.

15. Ines Wagner, "How Iceland Is Closing the Gender Wage Gap," *Harvard Business Review,* January 8, 2021, https://hbr.org/2021/01/how-iceland-is-closing-the-gender-wage-gap.

16. Íris Ellenberger, "The Day Women Brought Iceland to a Standstill," *Jacobin,* October 24, 2019, https://jacobinmag.com/2019/10/iceland-redstockings-womens-strike-feminism.

17. Verónica Gago, *Feminist International: How to Change Everything* (New York: Verso, 2020),185.

18. Federici, *Revolution at Point Zero*, 16.
19. Johnnie Tillmon, "Welfare Is a Women's Issue."

Chapter 3: Mothering as Erotic Labor

1. Viet Thanh Nguyen, "Failing Better: A Conversation with Ocean Vuong," *Los Angeles Review of Books*, June 24, 2019, https://lareviewofbooks.org/article/failing-better-a-conversation-with-ocean-vuong/.
2. Claudia Tate, ed., "Audre Lorde," *Black Women Writers at Work* (New York: Continuum, 1983), 100–16.
3. Lorde, "Uses of the Erotic," 53.
4. Lorde, "Uses of the Erotic," 54.
5. Mierle Laderman Ukeles, "Maintenance Art," Manifesta 10, September 28, 2014, https://www.youtube.com/watch?v=2k_twLupm8Y.
6. Mierle Laderman Ukeles, "Manifesto for Maintenance Art," 1969, https://www.queensmuseum.org/wp-content/uploads/2016/04/Ukeles_MANIFESTO.pdf.
7. Jillian Steinhauer, "How Mierle Laderman Ukeles Turned Maintenance Work into Art," *Hyperallergic*, February 10, 2017, https://hyperallergic.com/355255/how-mierle-laderman-ukeles-turned-maintenance-work-into-art/.
8. Mierle Laderman Ukeles, "For → Forever," Queens Museum of Art, 2020, https://queensmuseum.org/2020/09/mierle-laderman-ukeles.
9. Ukeles, "Manifesto for Maintenance Art."
10. She's referring to a a biblical story: "As Jesus and his disciples were on their way, he came to a village where a woman named Martha opened her home to him. She had a sister called Mary, who sat at the Lord's feet listening to what he said. But Martha was distracted by all the preparations that had to be made. She came to him and asked, 'Lord, don't you care that my sister has left me to do the work by myself? Tell her to help me!' 'Martha, Martha,' the Lord answered, 'you are worried and upset about many things, but only one thing is needed. Mary has chosen what is better, and it will not be taken away from her.' Source: https://www.bibleodyssey.org/en/people/main-articles/mary-and-martha.

11. Marge Piercy, "To Be of Use," *Circles on the Water* (New York: Knopf, 1982), 106.

12. "Atlanta's Washerwomen Strike," AFL-CIO, https://aflcio.org /about/history/labor-history-events/atlanta-washerwomen -strike.

13. Tera W. Hunter, *To 'Joy My Freedom: Southern Black Women's Lives and Labors After the Civil War* (Harvard University Press), 1997.

14. Angela Davis, "The Approaching Obsolescence of Housework: A Working-Class Perspective," *Women, Race, and Class* (New York: Vintage Books, 1983), 378, 392.

Chapter 4: Mothering as Human Interdependence

1. Luis H. Francia, *A History of the Philippines: From Indios Bravos to Filipinos* (New York: Overlook Press, 2014), 34.

2. Francia, *A History of the Philippines*, 34.

3. Patel and Moore, *A History of the World in Seven Cheap Things*, 128.

4. Kathryn Jezer-Morton, "What It Was Like Growing Up on a Commune," *The Nation*, March 6, 2021, https://www.thenation .com/article/society/commune-parenting-radical-community/.

5. Double Shift Interview with Dani McClain, October 15, 2020.

6. Hong, *Minor Feelings*, 86.

7. Mia Birdsong, *How We Show Up: Reclaiming Family, Friendship, and Community* (New York: Hachette, 2020), 17–18.

8. Dada Docot, May 25, 2021, https://twitter.com/dadadocot /status/1397430345687986179?s=20.

9. Patricia Hill Collins, "The Meaning of Motherhood in Black Culture and Black Mother-Daughter Relationships," *Sage*, vol. 4, issue 2, Fall 1987, 4.

10. Collins, "The Meaning of Motherhood in Black Culture and Black Mother-Daughter Relationships," 4.

11. Collins, "The Meaning of Motherhood in Black Culture and Black Mother-Daughter Relationships," 4.

12. Double Shift interview with Andrea Landry, March 9, 2021.

13. Mary Pipher, *Women Rowing North: Navigating Life's Currents and Flourishing as We Age* (New York: Bloomsbury, 2019), 31.

14. Carvell Wallace, "Trying to Parent My Black Teenagers Through Protest and Pandemic," *New York Times Magazine*, June 15, 2020,

https://www.nytimes.com/2020/06/15/magazine/parenting
-black-teens.html.

Chapter 5: Mothering Insists on Worthiness

1. World Health Organization, "World Report on Disability Fact-
    sheet," 2011, https://cdn.who.int/media/docs/default-source
    /documents/disability/world-report-on-disability-factsheet.pdf.
2. Centers for Disease Control and Prevention, "Disability Im-
    pacts All of Us," https://www.cdc.gov/ncbddd/disabilityand
    health/infographic-disability-impacts-all.html.
3. Sara Hendren, *What Can a Body Do? How We Meet the Built World*
    (New York: Riverhead Books, 2020), 14.
4. Sunaura Taylor, *Beasts of Burden: Animal and Disability Liberation*
    (New York: New Press, 2017), 16.
5. Hendren, *What Can a Body Do?*, 14.
6. Hendren, *What Can a Body Do?*, 32.
7. Pipher, *Women Rowing North*, 30.
8. Leah Lakshmi Piepzna-Samarasinha, *Care Work: Dreaming Disabil-
    ity Justice* (Vancouver, BC, Canada: Arsenal Pulp Press, 2018), 28.
9. Taylor, *Beasts of Burden*, 17.
10. Judy Heumann, *Being Heumann: An Unrepentant Memoir of a Dis-
    ability Rights Activist* (Boston, MA: Beacon Press, 2020), 113–14.
11. Nicole Newnham and Jim LeBrecht, directors, *Crip Camp*, 2020.
12. Piepzna-Samarasinha, *Care Work*, 78.
13. Piepzna-Samarasinha, *Care Work*, 78.
14. Hendren, *What Can a Body Do?*, 97–101.
15. Hendren, *What Can a Body Do?*, 45–46.
16. Neil Marcus, *Storm Reading*, 1988. See also Taylor, *Beasts of Bur-
    den*, 136.
17. Taylor, *Beasts of Burden*, 136.
18. Tina Cho, *The Ocean Calls: A Haenyeo Mermaid Story* (New York:
    Kokila, 2020).
19. Pipher, *Women Rowing North*, 30.

Chapter 6: Mothering as Encouraging Appetites

1. Carmen Maria Machado, "The Trash Heap Has Spoken," *Guer-
    nica*, February 13, 2017, https://www.guernicamag.com/the
    -trash-heap-has-spoken/.

2. Virginia Sole-Smith, *The Eating Instinct: Food Culture, Body Image, and Guilt in America* (New York: Henry Holt and Company, 2018), 234.

3. Tressie McMillan Cottom, "In the Name of Beauty," *Thick* (New York: The New Press, 2019), 71.

Chapter 7: Mothering Toward Movement

1. David Goode, *A World Without Words: The Social Construction of Children Born Deaf and Blind* (Philadelphia, PA: Temple University Press, 2010), 35.

2. Taylor, *Beasts of Burden*, 136–37.

3. Gia Kourlas, "Bill T. Jones Knows Life Will Change, and His Art Too," *New York Times*, May 20, 2020, https://www.nytimes.com/2020/05/20/arts/dance/bill-t-jones-deep-blue-sea-virus.html.

4. Alyx Gorman and Brigid Delaney, "Broadside 2019: How a Feminist Festival Took on Feminism—and Forced Us to Think Harder," *Guardian*, November 10, 2019, https://www.theguardian.com/culture/2019/nov/11/broadside-2019-how-a-feminist-festival-took-on-feminism-and-forced-us-to-think-harder.

5. Bessel van der Kolk, *The Body Keeps the Score* (New York: Penguin, 2004), 3.

6. Christine Caldwell, "Body Identity Development: Who We Are and Who We Become," from Christine Caldwell and Lucia Bennet Leighton, eds., *Oppression and the Body: Roots, Resistance, and Resolutions* (Berkeley, CA: North Atlantic Books, 2018), 42–43.

7. Rebecca Solnit, *Wanderlust: A History of Walking* (New York: Penguin, 2000), 10.

8. Global Health and Fitness Association, "2021 IHRSA Global Report," https://www.ihrsa.org/publications/the-2021-ihrsa-global-report/.

9. Isobel Asher Hamilton, "The CEO of Exercise-Bike Startup Peloton Says the Company 'Sells Happiness' in His Big Pitch to Investors," *Business Insider*, August 28, 2019, https://www.businessinsider.com/peloton-ceo-sells-happiness-more-than-bikes-2019-8.

10. Caldwell, *Bodyfulness: Somatic Practices for Presence, Empowerment, and Waking Up in This Life* (Boulder, CO: Shambhala, 2018), 14.

11. Piepzna-Samarasinha, *Care Work*, 72.
12. Anne Helen Petersen, "Against Kids' Sports," *Culture Study*, September 12, 2021, https://annehelen.substack.com/p/against -kids-sports.
13. Galen Cranz, *The Chair: Rethinking Culture, Body, and Design* (New York: W. W. Norton, 2000), 23.
14. Hendren, *What Can a Body Do?*, 75.
15. Cranz, *The Chair*, 23.
16. Tomer Heymann, director, *Mr. Gaga: A True Story of Love and Dance*, 2017.
17. Caldwell, *Bodyfulness*, 32–33.

Chapter 8: Mothering for Pleasure

1. Peggy Orenstein, *Girls & Sex: Navigating the Complicated New Landscape* (New York: HarperCollins, 2016), 71.
2. Orenstein, *Girls & Sex*, 62.
3. Guttmacher Institute, "Sex and HIV Education," October 1, 2021, https://www.guttmacher.org/state-policy/explore/sex -and-hiv-education.
4. Jennifer S. Hirsch and Shamus Khan, *Sexual Citizens: A Landmark Study of Sex, Power, and Assault on Campus* (New York: W. W. Norton, 2020), xvii.
5. Christina Cauterucci, "Ignorance Is Blessed," *Slate*, May 15, 2019, https://slate.com/news-and-politics/2019/05/alabama -abortion-law-republican-ignorance-female-reproduction.html.
6. A. Andrews, *A Quick & Easy Guide to Sex & Disability* (Portland, OR: Limerence Press, 2020), 24.
7. Piepzna-Samarasinha, *Care Work*, 72.
8. Luis H. Francia, *A History of the Philippines*, 42.
9. Bruce Bagemihl, *Biological Exuberance: Animal Homosexuality and Natural Diversity* (New York: St. Martin's Press, 1999), 18–19.
10. Esther Perel, *Mating in Captivity: Unlocking Erotic Intelligence* (HarperCollins, 2017), 41.

Chapter 9: Mothering as Natural Interdependence

1. Denise Levertov, "Sojourns in the Parallel World," from *Sands of the Well* (New York: New Directions, 1998).

2. Levertov, "Sojourns in the Parallel World."
3. Aldo Leopold, *A Sand County Almanac: And Sketches Here and There* (New York: Oxford University Press, 2020), 192.
4. Jenny Odell, *How to Do Nothing: Resisting the Attention Economy* (New York: Melville House, 2019), 183.
5. Solnit, *Wanderlust*, 10.
6. Odell, *How to Do Nothing*, 183.
7. Francia, *A History of the Philippines*, 44.
8. Robin Wall Kimmerer, "The Serviceberry: An Economy of Abundance," *Emergence Magazine*, December 10, 2020, https://emergencemagazine.org/essay/the-serviceberry/.
9. Kimmerer, "The Serviceberry."
10. Louise Clifton, "generations," reprinted in *Black Nature*, Camille T. Dungy, ed. (Athens, GA: University of Georgia Press), 57.
11. Wallace, "Trying to Parent My Black Teenagers Through Protest and Pandemic."

ABOUT THE AUTHOR

ANGELA GARBES is the author of *Like a Mother*, an NPR Best Book of the Year and finalist for the Washington State Book Award in nonfiction. Her work has appeared in the *New York Times*, *The Cut*, *New York*, *Bon Appétit*, and featured on NPR's *Fresh Air*. She lives with her family in Seattle.